AMERICAN INSTITUTE FOR ECONOMIC RESEARCH

# CORONAVIRUS AND DISEASE MODELING

EDITED BY

PETER C. EARLE

ISBN: 9781630692117

Cover art: Vanessa Mendozzi

# CORONAVIRUS AND DISEASE MODELING

EDITED BY
PETER C. EARLE

AIER | AMERICAN INSTITUTE *for* ECONOMIC RESEARCH

# CONTENTS

# INTRODUCTION

We live in a world inundated with, and crafted by, data. It's created, collected, gathered, stored, used, and often reused, alone or in conjunction with other data elements. It becomes an input for both simple decisions and in dauntingly complex models. But despite their nominal exactness, quantitative undertakings carry all of the same failings of the individuals and organizations that create, gather, and employ them. This is true of healthcare, the media, sports, finance, economics, gaming, and beyond.

We accept it as is. What else can we do?

To understand data inaccuracies and their implications, consider baseball.

It would have been just Yogi Berra's style to have said: "For a simple game, baseball is complicated." And he'd have been right: baseball is deceptively straightforward, with a handful of positions leading to a wide variety of strategies. And there are countless archaic and analytical approaches to player evaluation.[1] At the professional level,

---

1 Glassey, Connor. 2010. "What Are Baseball Scouts Looking For?" *Baseball America*, August 18; 2016. João de Carvalho. "Moneyball: Science vs scouts." *YouTube*, November 23.

the rewards are considerable for players, teams, and the cities that host them.[2] And for the season champions, the already-considerable rewards mount quickly.[3]

For these and other reasons, there is always some temptation to cheat. The most recent accusations involve alleged activities on the part of the Houston Astros—stealing signals between opposing catchers and pitchers and relaying them to batters—which took place during 2017, a point in time that coincides with their sudden shot to the top of certain rankings.[4] And additionally, there are suspicions that the alleged activity continued until recently.[5] Although ultimately bested by the Washington Nationals in the 2019 World Series, the Astros have been among the winningest teams in baseball over the last half decade.[6]

The accusations, still unproven, also cast doubt over other Astros

---

2 Fiorillo, Steve. 2019. "Who Are the Highest-Paid MLB Players in 2019?" *The Street*, March 1; Oznian, Mike, and Kurt Badenhausen. 2019. "Baseball Team Values 2019: Yankees Lead League At $4.6 Billion." *Forbes*, April 10; Uliano, Dick. 2019. "World Series could mean $6.5M to $8.8M for DC." *wtopnews*, October 16.

3 Elkins, Kathleen. 2019. "How much money the 2019 World Series champions will earn." *CNBC*, October 25.

4 Staszewski, Joseph. 2019. "Astros' emails reveal how deep cheating scandal went in 2017." *New York Post*, November 16; Jomboy (@Jomboy_). 2019. "Astros using cameras to steal signs, a breakdown." *Twitter*, November 12, 2019. https://twitter.com/LmgSTL/status/1194992074489311233.

5 Normandin, Marc. 2018. "The Astros have been cheating all season, maybe." *SBNation*, October 17; Fonseca, Brian. 2019. "MLB rumors: Is there proof Astros cheated vs. Yankees in 2019 ALCS?" *NJ.com*, November 18.

6 Wikipedia. 2020. "2019 Houston Astros season." *Wikipedia*, May 30; 2020. "Year-by-Year Results." *Astros.com*.

feats from the previous few seasons.[7] And where the team falls in terms of some of the more esoteric metrics is, frankly, astonishing.[8]

Now, it's true that cheating in baseball isn't new.[9] But as innocuous as it may seem, cheating casts a long shadow. Walking through the chain of causality, making batters more effective—which is to say, artificially boosting the data associated with hitting—immediately impacts on-base percentage (OBP) for both the players individually and the team overall.[10] In 2019, Houston also had the highest team batting average, slugging percentage, OPS, and was in the top three in runs, overall hits, home runs, total bases, and RBI.

Advantaged batters also negatively impact the statistics of the pitchers they face in several ways. With around 1,200 professional baseball players in any given season, and another 5,000 to 6,000 on minor league rosters, a handful of bad pitching performances owing to sign stealing can change a player's entire career trajectory.[11] And that's just cheating. The broader issue of inaccuracies and errors in baseball

---

7 Rome, Chandler. 2019. "Astros destroy Orioles with 23 runs to set franchise record." *Houston Chronicle*, August 10; Murray, Brian. 2019. "Astros: This season's offense may be the best in team history." *Climbing Tal's Hill*, October. Kram, Zach. 2019. "The Astros Have Brought the Murderers' Row Lineup Back to Baseball." *The Ringer*, October 4.

8 Sawchik, Travis (@Travis_Sawchik). 2019. Reply to @Jonathan-Drake. *Twitter*, November 12, 2019. https://twitter.com/JonathanDrake/status/1194362896056107008

9 The Week Staff. 2007. "Baseball's cheating heart." *The Week*, January 1; Wikipedia. 2020. "Black Sox Scandal." *Wikipedia*, May 25; Wikipedia. 2020. "Pine Tar Incident." *Wikipedia*, June 1.

10 Whether or not the alleged cheating is the cause, the Houston Astros had the highest OBP this year.

11 Slowinski, Steve. 2010. "Whip." *FanGraphs*, February 17.

officiating has come under scrutiny in recent years, and by dint of one of the most common agents nowadays: technology.[12]

By one estimation, umpires make almost 35,000 errors in a single season—an average of 14 mistakes per game—which, like the alleged cheating described earlier, immediately flow through performance data to skew game outcomes, distort players' career records, and further down the line impact fan experiences, wagers, and nearly every other aspect of the game.[13] Research shows that at certain ball/strike counts, umpires tend to favor pitchers over batters; that there are places within the strike zone that umpires tend to call wrong more than others (between 2008 and 2018, pitches to the top right and left portions of the strike zone were called incorrectly 27% of the time); and stranger still, that younger, less experienced umpires make better calls than older, more experienced ones. By other accounts, umpires often make calls that are decidedly biased in favor of the home team.[14]

But this is not where it ends. Beyond the earnings of teams and the career prospects of players, the influence of sabermetrics on scouting decisions and millions of bettors placing billions of dollars worth of real and fantasy sports wagers are subsequently influenced, mostly

12 Cortez, Julio. 2019. "'Robot umpires' in baseball have officially arrive." *MarketWatch*, July 11.

13 Williams, Mark T. 2019. "MLB Umpires Missed 34,294 Ball-Strike Calls in 2018. Bring on Robo-umps?" *BU Today*, April 8. Foreseeably the umpire's union, which has itself come under scrutiny at times, is not especially welcoming of the robo-umpires. See: Sanchez, Sara. 2019. "The MLB Umpires Association is a flawed and opaque organization." *Bleed Cubbie Blue*, June 19.

14 Briggs, Dave. 2016. "The next job at risk of being marginalized by robots: Major League Baseball's umpires." *CNBC*, October 31.

in negative ways.[15] The effects ripple further still, to sports agents, endorsement deals, and merchandisers: all, to some extent or another, influenced by the knock-on effects of faulty data.

Not very long ago, erroneous or misleading statistics could only do so much harm, but after the Moneyball revolution, quantitative analysis is a major part of how the business of baseball is conducted:[16]

> In 2003, there were maybe four to five clubs that had analytics-dedicated people on their payroll, and typically they were in an office down the hall working on recommendations to people who may or may not pay any attention.[17] I think what's changed today is that every general manager has some background or interest in analytics, and the typical size of the group in the front office is probably somewhere between 12 and 15 full-time people who all have advanced degrees, whether it's computer science or physics or mathematics or some other discipline. Along with that, there are data departments in organizations. Most organizations now have database folks and data scientists that are on their payroll and that are helping them not only store the information and organize it properly but also evaluate what it means.

---

15 Purdum, David. 2016. "A record $1 billion bet on MLB in 2016." *ESPN*, December 6; Gouker, Dustin. 2019. "Draftkings Does Deal with MLB to Become An 'Authorized Gaming Operator'." *Legal Sports Report*, July 25.

16 Lewis, Michael. 2003. *Moneyball: The Art of Winning an Unfair Game.* W.W. Norton & Co.: New York.

17 2018. "A view from the front lines of baseball's data-analytics revolution." *McKinsey & Company*, Interview, July 5.

For this reason, imprecise metrics—whether borne of cheating, erroneous calls, or subjective judgments—have both short- and long-term consequences of a systemic nature.[18] It is not unduly dramatic to suggest that somewhere, each year, a handful (or more) of great players who might have been drafted or called up from the minors to the majors are overlooked due to the direct or indirect effects of inaccurate data or faulty calculations. A veritable cascade of mislaid, invisible consequences thus propagates throughout the entire baseball ecosystem for years to come, mistakes perpetuated through historical databases and the memories of decision-makers.

Now: does anyone doubt that the US economy, indeed any economy (even a virtual economy), is vastly more complex than baseball? In 1963, Oskar Morgenstern published a 2nd edition of *On the Accuracy of Economic Observations*, in which he took to task the growing complacency with which economic data, in particular that which is tracked, compiled, analyzed, and released by governments, was increasingly regarded.[19] Noting that the growth of computing and the spread of econometrics were rapidly lending a physical science sheen to what is fundamentally a social science, he outlined the common problems with economic statistics (purposeful misrepresentations, errors, lack of definition, problems of classification, an inability to design experiments, bespoke interpretations, inappropriate aggregations, and so on) as they manifest in several areas: foreign trade, prices, unemployment,

---

18 Davis, Ryan. 2018. "25 Baseball Players Who Were Caught Cheating." *SportsCasting*, April 28; League Bat. 2014. "Worst Call in Major LEague Baseball History." *YouTube*, July 31. Marche, Stephen. 2017. "The Error in Baseball and the Moral Dimension to American Life." *The New Yorker*, October 2.

19 Morgenstern, Oskar. 1963. *On the Accuracy of Economic Observations*. 2nd Ed. Princeton University Press.

national income, and growth rates.

The very least that could and should be done, Morgenstern concluded, is (somewhat ironically) to emulate the physical sciences, albeit in one of its decidedly less glamorous habits: prominently displaying error estimates alongside all economic data releases.

> Perhaps the greatest step forward that can be taken, even at short notice, is to insist that economic statistics be only published together with an estimate of their error. Even if roughly estimated this would produce a wholesome effect. Makers and users of economic statistics must both refrain from making claims and demands that cannot be supported scientifically. The publication of error estimates would have a profound influence upon the whole situation … [Economists and students] must be brought up in an atmosphere of healthy distrust of the "facts" put before them. They must also learn how terribly hard it is to get good data and found [sic] out what really is "a fact."

Big data and the consequent analytical methods have certainly found their way into the planning and designs of the Federal Reserve System, the United State Department of the Treasury, the Bureau of Labor and Statistics, and other repositories of economic statistics.[20] They have also figured prominently into the government response to

---

20 Brave, Scott A., R. Andrew Butters, and David Kelley. 2019. "A New "Big Data" Index of U.S. Economic Activity." *Federal Reserve Bank of Chicago, Economic Perspectives,* 43(1); Heckman, Jory. 2019. "Treasury Dept. to overhaul CFO role with focus on data-driven decision-making." *Federal news Network,* September 2; Konny, Crystal G., Brendan K. Williams, and David M. Friedman. 2019. "Big Data in the U.S. Consumer Price Index: Experiences and Plans." *NBER.*

the ongoing pandemic, and often with pernicious results. This book focuses upon those: while the patina of state expertise often gives the reporting body the "benefit of the doubt" with respect to data integrity and quality, a bit more skepticism is in order.[21] There is plenty of reason to doubt the quality of government data and modeling, whether of its own production or compiled from outside sources.[22]

Consider that in December of 2018, the Federal Reserve raised the target range of its benchmark (Federal Funds) rate from 2.25% to 2.50%.[23]

> On July 31, the Federal Reserve cut the federal funds by 25-basis points to a range of 2% to 2¼%, and announced that it ended "quantitative tightening" immediately, two months before the scheduled end. The FOMC gave fuzzy guidance on future cuts, which sets up stock market uncertainties … The Fed under the orchestration of Fed Chair Jerome Powell has been flip-flopping, which has questioned FOMC independence and transparency.

And more recently, at least according to the President, discussions

---

21 Federal Reserve. 2019. "Dodd-Frank Act Stress Test 2019: Supervisory Stress Test Methodology March - 2019." *Federal Reserve*, April 9.

22 LSTA. 2018. "Slight SOFR SNAFU *But Rate Barely Moves)." *LSTA*, April 19; Hansen, Steven. 2010. "February Economic Data Enters the Bermuda Triangle." *Seeking Alpha*, March 21; Bennett, Robert A. 1979. "Manufacturers Hanover Concedes It Erred on Money Supply Figures." *The New York Times*, October 27; Wells, Rob. 1993. "Mozer Pleads Guilty to Falsifying Treasury Bids." *AP News*, October 1; Mantell, Ruth. 2015. "Here are the staff forecasts that the Fed accidentally leaked." *MarketWatch*, July 24.

23 Cox, Jeff. 2018. "Fed hikes rate, lowers 2019 projection to 2 increases." *CNBC*, December 19.

have included negative interest rates. If the Fed, with its massive troves of economic and financial data, untold sums of computing power, and veritable hordes of Ph.D economists, statisticians, and computer scientists find reason to completely reverse direction—whether driven by or in spite of data—any and all observers or users of said information should take pause.[24]

Oskar Morgenstern summarized his findings: "[T]he statistical problems of the social sciences cannot possibly be less serious than those of the natural sciences ... the situation is far more complicated and requires the most detailed scrutiny." But long before considerations regarding data quality, error estimates, and making sober assumptions: a heavy dose of humility is in order. The designers of epidemiological models would do well to emulate the words - actual, this time - of the always-sagacious Yogi Berra: "If you ask me something I don't know, I'm not going to answer."

The success that this project has had over the course of now three books would not have been possible without the considerable efforts of Alexander Gleason; thank you, Alex. David Schatz and Micha Gartz played key roles as well. Many (and I mean *many*) early morning, weekend, late night, and virtual conversations with Jeffrey Tucker, AIER's Editorial Director, were instrumental to maintaining momentum. And as the President of AIER, Edward Stringham provided both the leadership and intellectual environment which proved pivotal toward maintaining our focus amid fear-mongering and misinformation. And last but certainly not least, to Mary.

**Peter C. Earle**

August 3, 2020

---

24 Suttmeier, Richar Henry. 2019. "What's Up With Federal Reserve Policy." *Forbes*, August 12.

# THE LUDIC FALLACY

ˈ**lü-dik** ˈ**fa-lə-sē**, *n.* 1. Mistaking the well-posed problems of mathematics and laboratory experiments for the ecologically complex real world. Includes mistaking the randomness in casinos for that in real life.

## WORLD OF WARCRAFT'S CORRUPTED BLOOD OUTBREAK IS NOT A MODEL FOR COVID-19

BY PETER C. EARLE

May 28, 2020

On September 13, 2005, Blizzard Entertainment released Patch 1.7 for its still-young MMO game World of Warcraft.[1] Titled "Rise of the Blood God," it featured a series of new challenges and missions for players. And chief among those was a temple called Zul'Gurub containing a particularly nasty boss meant to challenge higher level players: the serpent-like demon god Hakkar the Soulflayer.[2] A description of the game lore is unnecessary (there's plenty of information available if you're interested), but for one detail: Hakkar was equipped with a particular nasty attack known as the Corrupted Blood spell.[3]

But whereas many attacks in games simply deal damage to players, Corrupted Blood had two fairly new tweaks. In addition to doing initial damage to the player, the spell was a debuff: it would continue to deal damage once every few seconds, slowly wearing down a player's health.[4] It was also designed to be "contagious," spreading

---

1 WoW. 2005. "Rise of the Blood God: Patch 1.7." *World of Warcraft*, September; Wikipedia. 2020. "Massively multiplayer online game." *Wikipedia*, July 17; Wikipedia. 2019. "World of Warcraft." *Wikipedia*, November 11.

2 WoWPedia. 2020. "Zul'Gurub (Classic)." *WoWPedia*, May 12; Wikipedia. 2020. "Boss (video games)." *Wikipedia*, July 6; Platinum Wow. 2020. "Zul'Gurub Classic WoW Guide DUNGEON DIVES." *YouTube*, April 4; WoWPedia. 2020. "Hakkar the Soulflayer." *WoWPedia*, June 22.

3 WoWPedia. 2020. "Zandalari Empire." *WoWPedia*, July 19; WoWPedia. 2020. "Corrupted Blood (debuff)." *WoWPedia*, April 18.

4 Wikipedia. 2019. "Status effect." *Wikipedia*, December 21.

from attacker to attacker, consequently forcing players to spread out during their assault on Zul'Gurub. An "infected" player could spread it to another in close proximity, that player could spread it to another, and so on.

Because the Corrupted Blood incident occurred shortly after the initial introduction of Patch 1.7, it's likely that one of the very first 20-player parties attempting to take on Hakkar in Zul'Gurub was responsible for the event which followed.

## A CONSEQUENTIAL OVERSIGHT

During the fight, some players must have noticed that the Corrupted Blood spell also infected pets.[5] And so to simplify the fight and reduce the distraction (and energy "cost") of healing both pets and characters, they dismissed them.[6]

As players emerged victorious from the Hakkar encounter—as is frequently the case in many fantasy MMOs—their first destination would typically be the game's major urban centers: specifically, markets.[7] There, they would sell some of the loot they'd won, repair damaged weapons and gear, and engage in social activities.[8] Unsurprisingly, markets are at any given time among the most densely populated areas of World of Warcraft.[9] And having dismissed their pets during the Hakkar battle, upon their return to cities and marketplaces many players called them back.

---

5 Pets are animal minions which accompany some characters into battle

6 Dismissing temporarily frees a pet, which can be called back later.

7 WoWPedia. 2020. "Auction House." *WoWPedia*, February 22.

8 WoWHead. 2019. "New Player Guide: Social Features in World of Warcraft." *WoW Head*, April 1.

9 And, in fact, most MMOs.

One can be reasonably certain that the development teams at Blizzard Entertainment were familiar with the concept of contagion and intended for the Corrupted Blood spell and its contagion to be limited to the instance within which the Hakkar the Soulflayer mission took place. But unbeknownst to players and developers alike, while the Corrupted Blood disease was removed when players left Zul'Gurub... it stayed active on players' dismissed pets.

## THE INITIAL OUTBREAK

As pets were summoned back to masters in the densely-crowded virtual marketplaces, players immediately began contracting Corrupted Blood. And because the difficulty of the Hakkar encounter was reflective of the skill and strength of the high-level characters that it was intended to attract, Corrupted Blood was a particularly dangerous spell: a serious annoyance for high-level characters, but devastating and often instantly lethal to lower-level players. Some players with enough health to not be instantly killed ran out of the marketplaces into other areas of the city; others—some infected, some not—quickly teleported elsewhere. Corrupted Blood was soon racing through numerous World of Warcraft cities and towns all across the virtual world, spreading and killing scores of characters representing tens or even hundreds of thousands of human players. Meanwhile, players in areas far-flung from marketplaces or cities teleported closer to observe the growing panic, increasing both the virtual body count and in some cases furthering its spread.

## PANDEMONIUM

Some players initially thought that what they saw occurring was a prank or an unannounced Blizzard marketing event. But for others, the rapidity and indiscriminate spread of the Corrupted Blood led to the conclusion that they were witnessing the unfolding of an unintended disaster.

As information about the Corrupted Blood outbreak spread, some took action. Alone or with other players—some in groups already bound together by guilds, others spontaneously organized—some high-level players shepherded low-level, more vulnerable players out of cities to avoid the rapidly expanding plague. Players without healing abilities "yelled" updates: some warning healthy players nearby to stay out of World of Warcraft cities, others giving locations of safe (self-isolation) zones.[10]

Some of the most powerful, high-level players with healing spells (priests and shamans) bravely attempted to resurrect or heal dead or dying lower-level players for long enough that they could either escape from the cities or arrive in what amounted to virtual first aid areas. While many players were healed of Corrupted Blood long enough to reach the comparably safer digital wilderness, other resurrected players quickly became re-infected and died again, sometimes spreading the disease a bit further in the process. And even some of the most powerful healers ultimately succumbed to Corrupted Blood, surrounded by the afflicted while attempting to administer aid.

The player-coordinated response to the pandemic, hours (and perhaps longer) before World of Warcraft's game managers got

---

10 The choice of the "yell" command is particularly interesting, as among the three forms of communication, the "say" command has a low, local range, and the "general chat" is as wide as the entire zone. Using "say" would have been of no use other than to players in the very immediate vicinity, while communicating via general chat would have drawn players from every corner of the zone, immediately overwhelming the safe zone. But "yell," with an in-game range of roughly 400 meters, allowed players to inform others of both danger and safe havens nearby without bringing a frenzied rush from all corners of the map.

involved—perhaps before they even understood the dimensions of the virtual disaster—was voluntary, emergent, and with small groups of survivors gathering in the distant wilds of World of Warcraft, arguably effective.

## REGROUPING

For four days (Sept 13–16, 2005) the plague spread. And at some point news of the curiosity—which certain World of Warcraft players were still certain was an intentional, global event—spread to the real world. Consequently, casual players logged in to watch the disease spreading "first hand;" some of them quickly getting infected, teleporting to other areas, and passing the Corrupted Blood to "healthy" players before expiring.

Survivors began communicating with friends, allies, and sometimes strangers in other regions of the game: relaying the locations of safe zones and attempting to piece together the source of the Corrupted Blood scourge. As they pieced together the pet-borne transmission element, a previously unknown piece of the puzzle fell into place: NPCs, non-player characters (thousands of whom "staff" markets and other important locations within the game) were spreading the disease as well, but did not bear any of the outward signs (a "splashing" effect). Thus NPCs were a particularly dangerous, if completely unintended, facet of the Corrupted Blood epidemic: asymptomatic carriers. And because NPCs cannot be killed, they stood as persistent carriers of Corrupted Blood. Having determined that, further announcements were made via general chat, travelling game-wide: despite their lack of outward appearance, players were warned, assume that all NPCs are infected with Corrupted Blood.

And as always with a highly social game (and no fear of ultimate mortality), a number of griefers took advantage of the fear and confusion: purposely infecting themselves with Corrupted Blood and searching for pockets of uninfected players.[11]

## CULMINATION

Major cities were all but abandoned, with some groups of players hiding out in dungeons (ironically, now some of the safest places in the game) or migrating toward less populated areas. By one account, the initial plague broke out in Ironforge; some survivors fled to Lakeshire, and others to Crossroads; then to the pirate haven of Booty Bay or Gadgetzan; and finally (again, ironically) many individuals and groups hunkered down in the unsettled, desolate region known as the Plaguelands.

At roughly 7:30am EST on September 16, 2005, a player posted in a forum reporting a disease spreading through Orgrimmar; a video appeared several hours later. At roughly 1:15pm EST, a Blizzard staffer reported that the firm was "aware of the issue and working on it."

Because of the ability of players to resurrect and be resurrected, and thus the possibility for the disease to spread without end—as opposed to real world outcomes including herd immunity, vaccine development, or darker (and unlikely) eschatological outcomes—the only solution was for game managers to reboot the servers: removing the Corrupted Blood infections all across the game world and modifying the Corrupted Blood spell code; the latter to no longer affect pets, and ensure in any case that the virtual disease could not leave the Hakkar

---

11 Wikipedia. 2020. "Griefer." *Wikipedia*, July 13.

encounter area.[12]

Ten hours later,[13] rolling restarts of the servers were announced, beginning at 7am EST on September 17th. The initial hotfix, applied during the rolling restarts, was unsuccessful, but after a second attempt the plague was stopped. The generally accepted time at which the Corrupted Blood plague ended was at just before 4pm EST on September 17th, 2005 after half a week of tumult and hundreds of thousands, perhaps millions, of character "deaths."

In the months and years after the incident, World of Warcraft's Corrupted Blood epidemic became a cause célèbre among certain scientists, including a handful of sociologists and epidemiologists. To be sure, World of Warcraft's Corrupted Blood episode makes a fascinating story. But to borrow from a memorable line, insofar as using it as a sociological, epidemiological, phenomenological, or in any sense as a model of human action under severe conditions: I come to bury the example of The Corrupted Blood, not to praise it.

## THE MODELING OBSESSION

There is a view that MMOs and other complex, large scale games may function as simulations of human behavior under extreme conditions, given that they involve the independent decisions of millions of players in a persistent space and thus effectively constitute a massive, computational petri dish.

To be sure, social science factors are missing from virtually all

---

12 Wikipedia. 2020. "Herd immunity." *Wikipedia*, July 2; Matheson, Richard. 1954. *I Am Legend*. Gold Medal Books: US; King, Stephen. 1978. *The Stand*. Doubleday: US.

13 About 11:30pm EST on September 16, 2005.

of the prevalent epidemiological models in use: regressions which, fed by historical data, current statistics, and certain environmental assumptions, trace a curve over time.[14] So too for agent-based models—models which populate a landscape with agents (each essentially an "individual" data structure with embedded characteristics and functions) and track their interactions over time—to predict infection, fatality, and other characteristics of spread of disease.[15] Epidemiological models which employ compartmental and network techniques are similarly bereft of social science elements.[16]

But examining the actions of game players and game designers or managers in the hope of gleaning anything more than expressly precise, superficial insights where behavior or policy making are concerned is self-deluding. In particular, casting game designers, developers, virtual community managers, and other decision makers of gaming firms as de facto governments, regulators, or central bankers is a woefully corrupt representation of the relationship between game players (consumers) and gaming firms (producers of for-profit ventures). As I have written previously,

---

14 Bender, Ralf. 2009. "Introduction to the use of regression models in epidemiology." *Methods in Molecular Biology*, 471: 179-195.

15 Perez, Liliana, and Suzana Dragicevic. 2009. "An agent-based approach for modeling dynamics of contagious disease spread." *International Journal of Health Geographics*, 8(50).

16 Brauer, Fred. 2008. "Compartmental Models in Epidemiology." *Mathematical Epidemiology,* 1945: 19-79; Keeling, Matt J., and Ken T.D. Eames. 2005. "Networks and epidemic models." *Journal of the Royal Society, Interface,* 2(4): 295–307.

> [w]hile their actions may ultimately generate similar outcomes, central planners seek and wield power whereas the actions of commercial gaming interests are undertaken to compete with other online entertainment providers by delicately balancing opportunities for newer players with the need to continually challenge experienced players.[17]

Actions undertaken by players in massive, multiplayer games may appear identical to those undertaken by living, breathing people, but draw from wholly different functions and motivations: game mechanics are at best a product of constrained choices in unique, virtual domains. Attempting to draw lasting, non-trivial conclusions to real-world problems from even the most complex games, wherein players face an entirely different set of opportunities, incentives, and epistemic conditions, is a fool's errand; although one for a sophisticated fool, to be sure.

Indeed: a paper airplane might briefly soar across a room the way a 747 does at 35,000 feet; but who would want to travel in the latter, if designed by the principles attending the former?

## CORRUPTED BLOOD IN THE AGE OF COVID-19

And predictably, since the start of the coronavirus crisis the assertion has been made that the 2005 Corrupted Blood incident could, or should, be considered a guide for addressing the spread of COVID-19. How?

Few laymen, let alone physicians, sociologists, economists, or

17 Earle, Peter C. 2013. "A Virtual Weimar: Hyperinflation in a Video Game World." *Mises Institute*, May 21.

epidemiologists, would be surprised that contagious diseases spread. Or that facing such a calamity, individuals may act heroically, idiotically, or even maliciously. Or that mistakes will be made. Would flesh-and-blood human beings be willing to live by policies derived from epidemiological studies on fantasy games? For example: one could argue that the strongest, highest-level healing characters did more harm than good by healing low-level infected players of the Corrupted Blood ailment who, in all likelihood, were going to die anyway; indeed, some of the weaker, rescued players lived long enough only to infect additional players before expiring anyway. Is the "lesson" that in a pandemic some citizens are beyond help and medical resources shouldn't be expended upon them? Or is the lesson that players in the game were somehow inadequately prepared for the disease outbreak, and thus that real-world governments should divert massive resources toward onshoring massive stockpiles of medicine, equipment and personal protective equipment in the face of unknown (and likely unknowable) future disease outbreaks?[18]

Consider the following comment from one academic paper. In Fall 2019—with the initial wave of COVID-19 infections only a month or two away—the *Berkeley Scientific Journal* reported that,

> [d]uring the initial phases of the [Corrupted Blood] epidemic, players, and later Blizzard Entertainment itself, established

---

18 AIER has written at length about the short-sighted, autarkic response to the spread of the novel coronavirus known as "medical-supply nationalism." See: Gulker, Max. 2020. "Medical-Supply Nationalism Is Deeply Harmful, Even Deadly." *American Institute for Economic Research*, March 20; Salter, Alexander W. 2020. "Can Medical Supply Autarky Save Us from Pandemics?" *American Institute for Economic Research*, April 19

> quarantines for characters to wait out the infection. Many players simply refused to obey the quarantine.[19]

Far more interesting than the idea of using a fantasy game as a model of the spread of a disease in the real world is a comment which seems to suggest a degree of incredulity at the notion that individuals, in any sense (and in particular, in a virtual, essentially riskless, entertainment venue) might not choose to stay put when and where ordered to.

People everywhere can be thankful, or perhaps hopeful, that this comment (from the same article) bears out and remains true:

> There have been many attempts to create a virtual world dedicated to social science and epidemiology research, with mixed success. Most manufactured worlds cannot hope to match the success of commercial MMOs, and most commercial MMOs do not have the time or motivation to work with epidemiologists without incentive.

## IF WE MUST DRAW LESSONS

The concept of using MMOs, incidentally or purposely, to plan epidemic (or any other disaster) policies confuses discoveries about gameplay with those regarding the actual, boundless choices, actions, and motivations of corporeal human beings under conditions of uncertainty and panic.

No, the Corrupted Blood event did not "perfectly predict" the

---

19 Girish, Nachiket. 2019. ""Corrupted Blood" and Public Health: What epidemiologists can learn from massively multiplayer video games." *Berkeley Scientific Journal*, Fall: 15-17.

outbreak and spread of the novel coronavirus.[20] No, the Corrupted Blood episode did not "teach us" how humans behave in outbreaks.[21] And no, video games will certainly not "rid the world" of COVID-19 or any other virus.[22] On the other hand, the Corrupted Blood outbreak in World of Warcraft was an excellent model, and provided highly relevant insights, as to how in Azeroth in 2005 fantasy game players would behave if a virulent, virtual plague suddenly appeared.

If we are bound to draw lessons—which may be another fool's errand—there are two that come to mind: one specifically for game developers, and one more broadly. Both come from Hayek.[23]

Drawing from Hayek's adage that "the curious task of economics is to demonstrate to men how little they really know about what they imagine they can design," modelers of real-world phenomena are well-reminded that in any complex system comprising numerous layers and connections, small changes in inputs lead to massive, often incomprehensible changes in output. Thus with the addition of another hundred, thousand, or million lines of new code; among hundreds, thousands, and millions of new objects, systems, and rules of virtual interaction; on top of the addition of another hundred, thousand, or million new players, the complexity of a social activity—and therefore of errors or unforeseen outcomes—increases, and in so doing becomes

---

20 Katwala, Amir. 2020. "World of Warcraft perfectly predicted our coronavirus panic." *Wired*, March 17.

21 Ouellete, Jennifer. 2020. "What a WoW virtual outbreak taught us about how humans behave in epidemics." *ARS Technica*, March 16.

22 McMahon, James. 2020. "Can video games help rid the world of COVID-19?" *NME*, April 30.

23 Econlib. n.d. "Friedrich August Hayek." *EconLib*.

increasingly difficult to predict. Which is to say: the real world, where individual human beings act, react and interact, is impossible to simulate.

To the second point, there is a conversation—again, in the spirit of Hayek—to be had regarding the way in which World of Warcraft players, shortly after the Corrupted Blood epidemic began, gathered and utilized relevant, actionable local information, employing it to guide arguably effective small-scale responses. Responses which, by nearly every account, facilitated responses long before Blizzard employees knew something unexpected was happening within the game.

But that conversation, and an apprehension of the factors at work there, is beyond models, computers, and social science supercolliders; it requires recognizing the existence and power of a social structure more complex than the human mind.[24] It is a conversation regarding the unsimulatable, a good start to which begins here: https://www.jstor.org/stable/1809376.[25]

---

24 Wikipedia. 2020. "Watson (computer)." *Wikipedia*, July 23; Ravindranath, Mohana. 2016. "DARPA Wants a 'Social Supercollider' To Help It Understand Humans." *NextGov*, September 9; Gulker, Max. 2019. "Markets Are More Complex Than Our Brains." *American Institute for Economic Research*, Marth 19.

25 Hayek, Friedrich A. 1945. "The Use of Knowledge in Society." *EconLib*.

## SIMCITY-STYLE MODELING FLUNKS THE REAL-WORLD TEST

BY PHILLIP W. MAGNESS

June 1, 2020

June 1st was supposed to mark a dreary milestone in the coronavirus pandemic. It is the day that the now-notorious Imperial College London (ICL) model predicted Sweden would peak at 95,000 COVID-19 deaths in the absence of a lockdown. In reality, Sweden currently sits at 4,395 deaths—a tragic loss to be certain, but also less severe than many other Western European nations under full lockdown.[25]

Sweden's shortfall from this expected death toll is good news for supporters of its comparatively mild and voluntary social distancing approach to the pandemic. But it also represents a complete failure of the predictive model that jarred much of the world including the United States and the United Kingdom into imposing draconian shelter-in-place policies that have now persisted for over two months.[26]

Back in early April, a team of epidemiologists at Uppsala University adapted the Imperial College model designed by crystal physicist Neil Ferguson to Sweden in an attempt to dissuade the country's government from its hands off approach.[27] Their results, like the more famous US

---

25 JHU. 2020. "COVID-19 Dashboard." *Johns Hopkins University*.

26 Landler, Mark, and Stephen Castle. 2020. "Behind the Virus Report That Jarred the U.S. and the U.K. to Action." *The New York Times*, March 17.

27 Gardner, Jasmine M., Lander Willem, Wouter Van Der Wijngaart, Shina Caroline Lynn Kamerlin, Nele Brusselaers, and Peter Kasson. 2020. " Intervention strategies against COVID-19 and their estimated impact on Swedish healthcare capacity." *medRxiv*, April 11; Ferguson, Neil M., Daniel Laydon, Gemma Nedjati-Gilani, Natsuko Imai, Kylie Ainslie et al. 2020. "Impact of non-pharmaceutical interventions (NPIs) to reduce COVID-19 mortality and healthcare demand." *Imperial College COVID-19 Response Team*, Report No. 9.

and UK iterations of the ICL model, predicted disaster if the country did not change course immediately.

A key graph from the study is depicted below, with markers to indicate where it was supposed to stand on June 1st. Point A represented what would happen if Sweden maintained its milder policies without a lockdown, yielding as many as 95,000 deaths. Point B shows their prediction for what would happen if Sweden changed course by April 10th and adopted a European-style lockdown similar to the strategy that their neighbors employed. As a relative latecomer to the lockdown game, Sweden would incur "only" 40,000 deaths by June 1st if its government fell into line with the rest of the world.

As it actually stands, Sweden sits at point C, well below either scenario and on a curve that was not even contemplated under the ICL model.

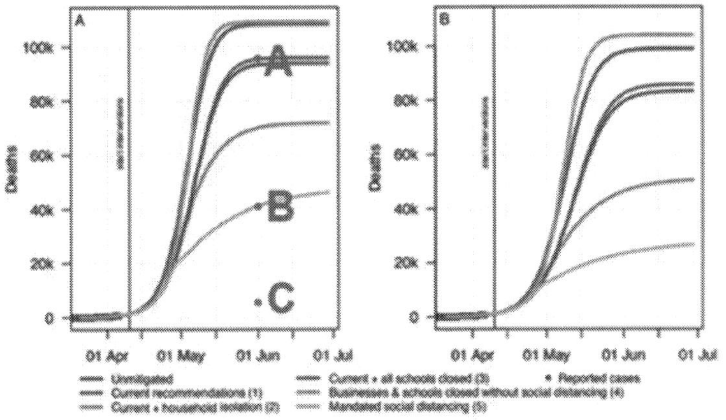


Figure 4. Estimated number of COVID-19 related deaths. Deaths are plotted for each public health intervention strategy over time, using models parameterized to doubling times of (A) 3 or (B) 5 days. For a description of each intervention modelled, see the Methods. Confidence intervals based on infection-fatality rates are listed in the text.

## HOW THE MODELERS WENT WRONG

Ferguson's ICL study is the most famous and influential example of a relatively recent type of epidemiology model known as an agent-based simulation.[28] Briefly summarized, the ICL approach purports to take known or approximated data about a virus's infection and fatality rates and subjects them to a simulation of expected transmission within a country or region, calibrated to its population characteristics and related demographic inputs.

The model then runs a succession of computer simulations that allegedly calculate how quickly the virus spreads given what they assume about the frequency of human social interactions. Since the models are probabilistic, they're usually carried out in repetition so the final result reflects multiple runs of the simulation.

To render the simulations useful for policymakers, modelers such as the ICL team then adjust their runs to account for a variety of proposed scenarios. While the first set of predictions might reflect a "do nothing" course of no interventions and an uncontrolled pandemic, a second scenario might include what they predict to happen if schools and large sporting events are closed. A third might predict adding voluntary social distancing to the mix. And a fourth might predict a full mandatory lockdown.

Under perfect knowledge of both a virus and human behavior in response to the virus and full understanding of how each affects transmission, a computer simulation of this type could at least—in theory—approximate an actual pandemic. Indeed, modelers such as Ferguson and the ICL team seem to believe they possess such

---

28 Adam, David. 2020. "Special report: The simulations driving the world's response to COVID-19." *Nature*, April 2.

knowledge and can accurately control for such complex scenarios to the point that it yields accurate predictive information about viruses.

In a sense it's an epidemiological approach that treats the world as a real-life version of the old SimCity computer game, and reports what happens if you play that game in repetition under the conditions of a pandemic.

The simulation approach has a severe deficiency though in that the assumptions and inputs it takes for granted are both unknown and sufficiently complex to render them unknowable.[29] Modelers have to fill in substantial gaps in their knowledge by imposing assumptions into their code—assumptions about the transmissibility of the virus, assumption about its duration and fatality rate, assumptions about the effectiveness of policy responses, and even assumptions about the rate that people will comply with or abide by those policies.

If we look to a key table from the ICL COVID model, we quickly find that these assumptions are little more than guesswork—particularly when it comes to the effectiveness of the proposed policy interventions. The table shows four modeled policy responses that purport to contain COVID-19. Note that all four adopt nice, even, round numbers as their parameters for modeling the proposed intervention: a 70% compliance rate with X, a 50% compliance rate with Y, and a 25% reduction in behavior Z, all allowing precise predictions of how the pandemic will supposedly play out.

---

29 Hayek, F.A. 1945. "The Use of Knowledge in Society." *The American Economic Review*, 35(4): 519-530.

**Table 2: Summary of NPI interventions considered.**

| Label | Policy | Description |
|---|---|---|
| CI | Case isolation in the home | Symptomatic cases stay at home for 7 days, reducing non-household contacts by 75% for this period. Household contacts remain unchanged. Assume 70% of household comply with the policy. |
| HQ | Voluntary home quarantine | Following identification of a symptomatic case in the household, all household members remain at home for 14 days. Household contact rates double during this quarantine period, contacts in the community reduce by 75%. Assume 50% of household comply with the policy. |
| SDO | Social distancing of those over 70 years of age | Reduce contacts by 50% in workplaces, increase household contacts by 25% and reduce other contacts by 75%. Assume 75% compliance with policy. |
| SD | Social distancing of entire population | All households reduce contact outside household, school or workplace by 75%. School contact rates unchanged, workplace contact rates reduced by 25%. Household contact rates assumed to increase by 25%. |
| PC | Closure of schools and universities | Closure of all schools, 25% of universities remain open. Household contact rates for student families increase by 50% during closure. Contacts in the community increase by 25% during closure. |

Curiously, there appears to be little effort in these models to test and verify whether the underlying assumptions are correct. They also do very little to account for behavioral changes during the course of the pandemic that will almost certainly alter factors such as compliance rates with policy directives, or even voluntary behaviors that people undertake on their own to mitigate the risks of the disease (think about increased hand-washing).[30] Instead, we have parameters that essentially amount to guesswork, all of it hard-coded into the model. And if any one of those underlying assumptions ends up being wrong, it

30 Aver, Christopher, William Bossert, Adam Clark, Glenn Ellison, and Sara Fisher Ellison. 2020. "Policy Implications of Models of the Spread of Coronavirus: Perspectives and Opportunities for Economists." *NBER*, Working Paper No. 27007.

potentially throws off the entire predictive ability of the model itself.

As the Swedish application of the ICL model reveals, one or more of its underlying assumptions about the coronavirus and the effectiveness of proposed policy interventions were clearly in error. Its predictions were therefore wholly implausible, and have already been invalidated by reality as the June 1st numbers demonstrate.[31]

In fact, we may see evidence that the ICL model was wholly unsuited to the coronavirus by looking into its history. Ferguson and the other ICL authors first developed this model in the mid-2000s as one of the two major contributions to the computer simulation approach for pandemics. The second came from a team led by Robert J. Glass, a modeler at the Los Alamos laboratory who adopted a similar approach.

Ferguson and Glass were both major figures in the epidemiology community's shift away from traditional disease-mitigation strategies and toward wide-scale lockdowns, as first proposed in 2006 following a succession of government research inquiries into influenza pandemics and the threat of bioterrorism.[32] The introduction of their modeling approach precipitated a debate among epidemiologists over the effectiveness of unproven strategies such as society-wide lockdowns, as well as lesser interventions such as school closures and event cancellations.[33]

Several figures in the medical wing of the discipline expressed doubts about top-down society-wide approaches such as lockdowns

---

31 Magness, Phillip W. 2020. "Imperial College Model Applied to Sweden Yields Preposterous Results." *American Institute for Economic Research*, April 30.

32 See article herein entitled "The 2006 Origins of the Lockdown Idea."

33 Glass, Robert J., Laura M. Glass, Walter E. Beyeler, and H. Jason Min. 2006. "Targeted Social Distancing Designs for Pandemic Influenza." *CDC Emerging Infectious Diseases*, 12(11).

at the time, noting the lack of empirical evidence behind the modeling assumptions as well as the complete absence of a causal identification strategy for the claimed effectiveness of its policy prescriptions. The modeling approach of Ferguson and Glass caught the ears of public health officials at the time though, and has since come to dominate the COVID-19 response.

Yet if we look back to Ferguson's original paper from 2006 in which he laid out the model that he later adapted to the current pandemic, we find another stunning revelation in its penultimate paragraph:[34]

> Lack of data prevent us from reliably modelling transmission in the important contexts of residential institutions (for example, care homes, prisons) and health care settings; detailed planning for use of antivirals, vaccines and infection control measures in such settings are needed, however. We do not present projections of the likely impact of personal protective measures (for example, face masks) on transmission, again due to a lack of data on effectiveness.

Among its many shortcomings, the original ICL model lacked a means of accounting for the transmission of viruses in residential institutions such as nursing homes and similar long-term care facilities. As the last several months have shown however, nursing homes are acutely susceptible to the coronavirus and may be the single largest

34 Ferguson, Neil M., Derek A.T. Cummings, Christophe Fraser, James C. Cajka, Philip C. Cooley, and Donald S. Burke. 2006. "Strategies for mitigating an influenza pandemic." *Nature*, 442: 448-452.

factor in explaining its high fatality rate.[35] In many countries and US states, nursing homes even account for more than half of all total coronavirus fatalities. In virus hotspots such as New York, the nursing home problem was compounded even further by likely undercounting deaths and an emergent scandal over Gov. Andrew Cuomo's order forcing nursing homes to admit known coronavirus carriers as a way of mitigating hospital capacity strains that were never actually realized.[36]

Returning to the question of epidemiology modeling, the nursing home issue may reveal a fatal flaw in the ICL model's underlying assumptions. If indeed it had no means of accounting for viral transmissions in residential institutions as Ferguson's 2006 paper indicates, the ICL model completely missed what now turns out to be the single greatest vulnerability point for the coronavirus pandemic.[37]

Such an oversight would further imply that the predictive scenarios of the ICL model's policy interventions are not only misdirected away from the primary vulnerability points and onto society at large, but also that the forecasted mortality ranges of its milder scenarios under the lockdown have little basis in reality.

If nursing homes account for the lion's share of COVID mortality as

---

35 Yourish, Karen, K.K. Rebecca Lai, Danielle Ivory, and Mitch Smith. 2020. "One-Third of All U.S. Coronavirus Deaths Are Nursing Home Residents or Workers." *The New York Times*, May 11.

36 McCaughey, Betsy. 2020. "New York's nursing home horrors are even worse than you think." *New York Post,* May 29; Associated Press. 2020. "AP count: Over 4,300 coronavirus patients sent to New York nursing homes." *Q13 Fox Seattle*, May 22.

37 The ICL team has thus far resisted calls to release its original code from the COVID simulation, and public versions of the same code are riddled with bugs and errors. The released version of its COVID paper does not give any indicator though that they modified the 2006 study to account for nursing homes

the statistics now show, the realized death rates in countries that went under lockdown may only be said to follow the ICL model's milder scenarios as a result of coincidence. Even when the total numbers in some countries appear to match up with the ICL's midler scenarios, the deaths predicted by the model are not the same types of deaths we are seeing in reality. When it comes to predicting the actual mechanisms of the pandemic, including the danger it poses to nursing homes, the modeling approach appears to be functionally useless and catastrophically off the mark.

## VISUALIZATIONS ARE POWERFUL, BUT OFTEN MISLEADING

BY JAMES L. CATON

May 14, 2020

Powerful data visualization can demonstrate in the blink of an eye what might take minutes, or even hours to uncover through reading and analysis. The power of visualization lies in the ability to quickly relate thousands or even millions of data points thereby conveying their meaning.

Each part of a visualization implies something. Very often I will plot lines. Depending on the nature of the visualization, meaning is conveyed by the slope or height of the line. A line whose values are increasing might show income increasing over time. Or, area under a curve might convey distance traveled if the units represented by the line are meters per second.

Very often, I will transform data to help clarify its meaning. In economics, it is common to take the logged value of data that is generated over time because logged values allow you to compare proportional change from one unit of time to the next. Suppose that your speed is consistently increasing so that it doubles every 10 seconds. Or imagine that your income doubles every year. Very quickly the value represented by the line will become quite large.

This is exemplified by a tale about the origins of chess. A king offered to reward the creator, who cleverly asked for a gift of rice (or wheat depending on the rendition) where for each square on the chess board, the number of grains would double, from 1 to 2, to 4, eventually reaching 263. Very quickly the king learned that he had failed to account for the magnitude of the gift! If we were to log the vertical axis to represent the story, the line used to represent the number of grains of rice for each additional square would be straight instead of becoming a rather steep curve. The slope of the line would approximate change as a percentage from one period to the next.

## COVID-19 DATA AND RULES OF THUMB FOR VISUALIZING DATA

As with any tool, visualization must be used responsibly. Tools for visualizing one type of data may not be appropriate for another. If I was to graph the speed of a car over time with the goal of indicating distance traveled, it would make little sense for me to log the vertical axis. For example, when I generate statistics for data, I do not log interest rates or estimate the percent change of an interest rate. I do calculate logged values and percent change for variables that are levels like real GDP and the quantity of dollars circulating in the U.S. economy.

To make improper transformation of data can lead observers of data to incorrect conclusions. As COVID-19 data has proliferated since the start of the year, I have observed time and time again individuals who present the data incorrectly. To name one pernicious sin, comparisons of the total number of cases or deaths between countries or between counties in the United States convey little to no information that is useful for comparing the state of spread in each entity. If the goal is to make inferences from comparison of data from different jurisdictions, then the data needs to control for population.

You must also consider the nature of a set of data. For example, even controlling for population, it makes little sense to compare the level of positive COVID-19 cases in countries that do not have comparable capacity to provide testing. The number of tests per million in the United States is going to be much higher than the number of tests per million in Afghanistan. These problems have been pervasive.

Today, I was surprised when I saw a new problem in the presentation of data concerning the state of the spread in Sweden. The *Financial Times* indicated that the daily number of deaths per million per day in Sweden recently passed that of Italy, UK, and Belgium. The article includes a graphic comparing the UK and Sweden and links to a graphic comparing Spain and Sweden.[38] Both visualizations used a logged y-axis to compare values that are already rates of change. As I have noted, the area under a curve indicates the accumulation of value over time in plots where the rate of change is indicated on the vertical axis and time on the horizontal axis.

If you log values represented by the vertical axis, this compresses the areas that are relatively large and expands the areas that are relatively small. The takeaway from the *Financial Times* article is somewhat ambiguous. The author does not take a hard stance one way or the other. The undertones of the article, however, are not ambiguous. This may not be the intention of the author, but the subtle details convey much.

The title of the article informs the reader that "Sweden's death toll unnerves its Nordic neighbors."[39] It cites data concerning differences of new deaths per million each day between Sweden, the U.K., Spain and Italy, but does not compare levels. It compares the level of total deaths per million in Sweden with the levels of its neighbors, Netherlands, Denmark and Norway.

38 Financial Times. 2020. "Coronavirus tracked: has the epidemic peaked near you?" *Financial Times*.

39 Financial Times. 2020. "Sweden's death toll unnerves its Nordic neighbours" *Financial Times*, May 20.

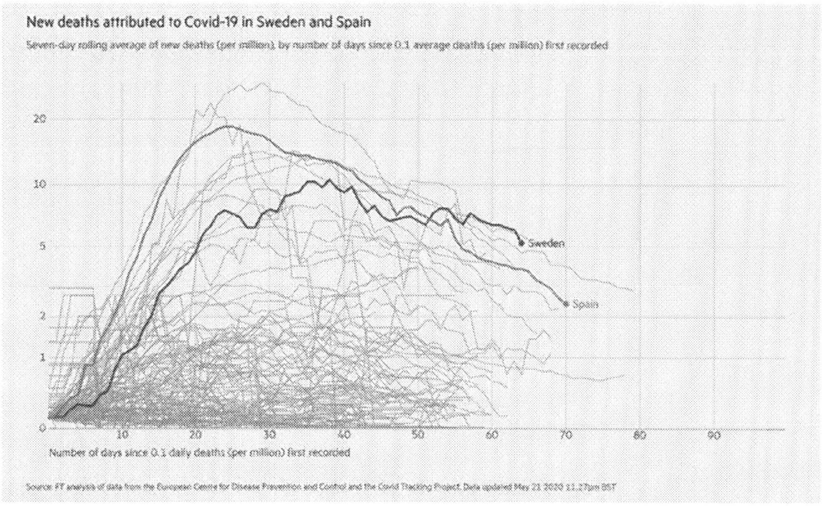


The article cites a politician from Denmark who is quite concerned:

> "I don't believe that Denmark should open its border to Sweden already because the COVID-19 situation is still out of control in Sweden. Denmark has to await a normalisation in Sweden. So this is a rational decision based only on the number of COVID-19 deaths," Peter Skaarup, parliamentary head of the populist Danish People's party, told the FT.

The perception among some in neighboring countries is that Sweden has adopted an extreme, and perhaps dangerous, policy.

I don't know exactly the sentiment that Sweden's neighbors in general hold toward its policy. The article may be truly representative on this front. However, I think it is appropriate to convey all of the facts, not just the negative. In this spirit, I offer the reader visualization comparing Sweden with other countries, highlighting Spain in particular. I present the data with logged vertical axes and unlogged vertical axes.

In the plots with unlogged values, the area beneath the curve represents the total number of COVID-19 related deaths in a country.

The area highlighted between curves represents the difference between Spain and Sweden. The reader will notice that the logged plots understate the level of deaths (area under the curve) for Spain relative to Sweden.

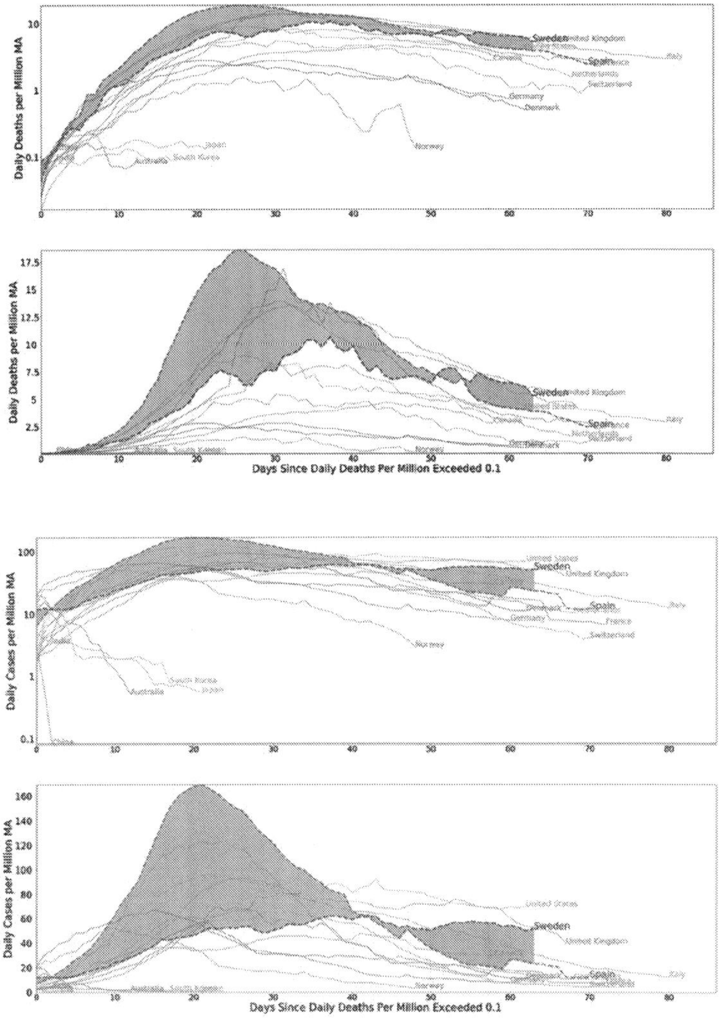

Sweden has flattened its curve without a lockdown on the presumption that the number of deaths that will result from its strategy will be on par with the number of deaths that would occur with a lockdown. Sweden's strategy has received praise from the WHO, but has received harsh criticism from some experts within the country.[40] Only time will tell if this assumption is correct.

My best guess—I am an economist, not an epidemiologist—is that we will not have the data necessary to judge until we see later waves of the spread. The epidemiologists that lead policy in Sweden are confident that their approach is the correct one.[41]

In light of my own preferences, I must recognize at least a few facts. Sweden's policy is not to minimize the rate of spread.[42] Their goal is to make the spread manageable, thereby limiting unnecessary loss of life. South Korea, on the other hand, has shown that a program of tracking from the earliest days of the spread is actually quite efficient at slowing the spread.

There is no comparison to the success that we've seen across Southeast Asia in slowing the spread. I'm more than a bit uncomfortable with a strategy that uses involuntary tracking to slow the spread, but its success is impossible to deny. Is the potential loss of liberty from growing surveillance worth bearing?

---

40 Ledel, Johannes. 2020. "As Europe Slowly Exits Lockdown, Sweden Hunkers Down for Long Haul." *Courthouse News Service*, May 20; Baker, Sinead. 2020. "Skeptical experts in Sweden say its decision to have no lockdown is a terrible mistake that no other nation should copy." *Business Insider*, May 21.

41 Dorroh, Jennifer. 2020. "Key quotes: Sweden's top epidemiologist challenges conventional wisdom on COVID-19." *International Journalists' Network*, May 11.

42 Weintraub, Karen. 2020. "Sweden Sticks With Controversial COVID-19 Approach." *WebMD*, May 1.

And although Sweden seems to be doing relatively well in light of the fact it has not locked down, it is being outperformed in terms of the level of deaths per million by a number of its neighbors who did lock down. Only time will tell if the end state will be different once a year or more has passed.

I also cannot hide that I am suspicious of policies that threaten liberty in the long-run and that appear to me to disrespect protections to our civil liberties provided by the U.S. Constitution. I'm uncomfortable with the fact that the virus has made us suspicious of one another. I look forward to a time that society returns to a higher level of openness.

I accept that a return to normalcy is part of democratic conversation that occurs fundamentally at the local level, and that many believe that every possible effort must be made to maximize the flattening of the curve. I must respect the concern of those around me. Most in the U.S. do not support a Sweden-type policy approach. I notice also that most are not comfortable discussing policy options.

While my interest drives the subject of my analysis, it should not categorically drive outcomes. I believe that democracy depends on a willingness to engage openly with ideas that challenge our fundamental beliefs and strongest preferences. If there exist a set of ideas that is strongly supported by evidence and that is at odds with my own beliefs, in the least I must respect the strength of the position, if not accept it altogether. I would be dishonest to do otherwise.

And, no matter my position, the data must be allowed to speak without being distorted. I leave it to the reader to interpret what it is saying.

## THE 2006 ORIGINS OF THE LOCKDOWN IDEA

BY JEFFREY TUCKER

May 15, 2020

Now begins the grand effort, on display in thousands of articles and news broadcasts daily, somehow to normalize the lockdown and all its destruction of the last two months. We didn't lock down almost the entire country in 1968/69, 1957, or 1949-1952, or even during 1918.[43] But in a terrifying few days in March 2020, it happened to all of us, causing an avalanche of social, cultural, and economic destruction that will ring through the ages.

There was nothing normal about it all. We will be trying to figure out what happened to us for decades hence.

How did a temporary plan to preserve hospital capacity turn into two-to-three months of near-universal house arrest that ended up causing worker furloughs at 256 hospitals, cessation of international travel, 40% job losses among people earning less than $40K per year, devastation of every economic sector, mass confusion and demoralization, the complete disregard of all fundamental rights and liberties, not to mention the mass confiscation of private property with forced

---

43 Tucker, Jeffrey A. 2020. "Woodstock Occurred in the Middle of a Pandemic." *American Institute for Economic Research*, May 1; Tucker, Jeffrey A. 2020. "Elvis Was King, Ike Was President, and 116,000 Americans Died in a Pandemic." *American Institute for Economic Research*, May 4; Tucker, Jeffrey A. 2020. "No Lockdowns: The Terrifying Polio Pandemic of 1949-52." *American Institute for Economic Research*, May 10; Geloso, Vincent. 2020. "Spanish Flu Was Awful But We Moved On Anyway." *American Institute for Economic Research*, April 14.

closures of millions of businesses?[44]

Whatever the answer, it's a bizarre tale. What's truly surprising is just how recent the theory behind lockdown and forced distancing actually is. So far as anyone can tell, the intellectual machinery that made this mess was invented 14 years ago, and not by epidemiologists but by computer-simulation modelers. It was adopted not by experienced doctors—they warned ferociously against it—but by politicians.

Let's start with the phrase social distancing, which has mutated into forced human separation. The first I had heard it was in the 2011 movie *Contagion*. The first time it appeared in the *New York Times* was February 12, 2006:[45]

> If the avian flu goes pandemic while Tamiflu and vaccines are still in short supply, experts say, the only protection most Americans will have is "social distancing," which is the **new politically correct way of saying "quarantine**."
>
> But distancing also encompasses less drastic measures, like wearing face masks, staying out of elevators—and the [elbow] bump. Such stratagems, those experts say, will rewrite the ways we interact, at least during the weeks when the waves of influenza are washing over us.

---

44 Paavola, Alia. 2020. "266 hospitals furloughing workers in response to COVID-19." *Becker's Hospital Review*, April 7; Tucker, Jeffrey A. 2020. "'I've Lost Faith in Humanity': The Psychological Toll of the Lockdown." *American Institute for Economic Research*, April 28.

45 McNeil, Donald G. Jr. 2006. "Greetings Kill: Primer for a Pandemic." *The New York Times*, February 12.

Maybe you don't remember that the avian flu of 2006 didn't amount to much. It's true, despite all the extreme warnings about its lethality, H5N1 didn't turn into much at all.[46] What it did do, however, was send the existing president, George W. Bush, to the library to read about the 1918 flu and its catastrophic results. He asked for some experts to submit some plans to him about what to do when the real thing comes along.

*The New York Times* tells the story from there:[47]

> Fourteen years ago, two federal government doctors, Richard Hatchett and Carter Mecher, met with a colleague at a burger joint in suburban Washington for a final review of a proposal they knew would be treated like a piñata: telling Americans to stay home from work and school the next time the country was hit by a deadly pandemic.
>
> When they presented their plan not long after, it was met with skepticism and a degree of ridicule by senior officials, who like others in the United States had grown accustomed to relying on the pharmaceutical industry, with its ever-growing array of new treatments, to confront evolving health challenges.
>
> Drs. Hatchett and Mecher were proposing instead that Americans in some places might have to turn back to an approach, self-isolation, first widely employed in the Middle Ages.
>
> How that idea—born out of a request by President George W.

---

46 CDC. 2018. "Highly Pathogenic Asian Avian Influenza A(H5N1) Virus." *CDC*, December 12.

47 Lipton, Eric, and Jennifer Steinhauer. 2020. "The Untold Story of the Birth of Social Distancing." *The New York Times*, April 22.

> Bush to ensure the nation was better prepared for the next contagious disease outbreak—**became the heart of the national playbook for responding to a pandemic** is one of the untold stories of the coronavirus crisis.
>
> It required the key proponents—Dr. Mecher, a Department of Veterans Affairs physician, and Dr. Hatchett, an oncologist turned White House adviser—to overcome intense initial opposition.
>
> It brought their work together with that of a Defense Department team assigned to a similar task.
>
> And it had some unexpected detours, including a deep dive into the history of the 1918 Spanish flu and an important discovery **kicked off by a high school research project pursued by the daughter of a scientist** at the Sandia National Laboratories.
>
> The concept of social distancing is now intimately familiar to almost everyone. But as it first made its way through the federal bureaucracy in 2006 and 2007, it was viewed as **impractical, unnecessary and politically infeasible**.

Notice that in the course of this planning, neither legal nor economic experts were brought in to consult and advise. Instead it fell to Mecher (formerly of Chicago and an intensive care doctor with no previous expertise in pandemics) and the oncologist Hatchett.

But what is this mention of the high-school daughter of 14? Her name is Laura M. Glass,[48] and she recently declined to be interviewed

48 A previous version of this article in one instance incorrectly named the coauthor of the 2006 paper by Robert Glass. That is now corrected to Laura M. Glass.

when the *Albuquerque Journal* did a deep dive of this history.[49]

> Laura, with some guidance from her dad, devised a computer simulation that showed how people—family members, co-workers, students in schools, people in social situations—interact. What she discovered was that school kids come in contact with about 140 people a day, more than any other group. Based on that finding, her program showed that in a hypothetical town of 10,000 people, 5,000 would be infected during a pandemic if no measures were taken, but only 500 would be infected if the schools were closed.

Laura's name appears on the foundational paper arguing for lockdowns and forced human separation. That paper is "Targeted Social Distancing Designs for Pandemic Influenza" (2006).[50] It set out a model for forced separation and applied it with good results backwards in time to 1957. They conclude with a chilling call for what amounts to a totalitarian lockdown, all stated very matter-of-factly.

> Implementation of social distancing strategies is challenging. They likely must be imposed for the duration of the local epidemic and possibly until a strain-specific vaccine is developed and distributed. If **compliance with the strategy is**

---

49 Reed, Ollie Jr. 2020. "Social distancing born in ABQ teen's science project." *Albuquerque Journal*, May 2.

50 Glass, Robert J., Laura M. Glass, Walter E. Beyeler, and H. Jason Min. 2006. "Targeted Social Distancing Designs for Pandemic Influenza." *CDC Emerging Infectious Diseases*, 12(11).

> **high** over this period, an epidemic within a community can be averted. However, if neighboring communities do not also use these interventions, infected neighbors will continue to introduce influenza and prolong the local epidemic, albeit at a depressed level more easily accommodated by healthcare systems.

In other words, it was a high-school science experiment that eventually became law of the land, and through a circuitous route propelled not by science but politics.

The primary author of this paper was Robert J. Glass, a complex-systems analyst with Sandia National Laboratories. He had no medical training, much less an expertise in immunology or epidemiology.

That explains why Dr. D.A. Henderson, "who had been the leader of the international effort to eradicate smallpox," completely rejected the whole scheme.

Says the *NYT*:

> Dr. Henderson was convinced that it made no sense to force schools to close or public gatherings to stop. Teenagers would escape their homes to hang out at the mall. School lunch programs would close, and impoverished children would not have enough to eat. Hospital staffs would have a hard time going to work if their children were at home.
>
> The measures embraced by Drs. Mecher and Hatchett would "result in significant disruption of the social functioning of communities and result in possibly serious economic problems," Dr. Henderson wrote in his own academic paper responding to their ideas.
>
> The answer, he insisted, was to tough it out: **Let the**

> **pandemic spread, treat people who get sick and work quickly to develop a vaccine to prevent it from coming back**.

AIER's Phil Magness got to work to find the literature responding to the 2006 paper by Robert and Laura M. Glass and discovered the following manifesto: "Disease Mitigation Measures in the Control of Pandemic Influenza."[51] The authors included D.A. Henderson, along with three professors from Johns Hopkins: infectious disease specialist Thomas V. Inglesby, epidemiologist Jennifer B. Nuzzo, and physician Tara O'Toole.

Their paper is a remarkably readable refutation of the entire lock-down model.[52]

The remarkable conclusion:

> Experience has shown that communities faced with epidemics or other adverse events respond best and with the least anxiety when the **normal social functioning of the community is least disrupted**. Strong political and public health leadership to provide reassurance and to ensure that needed medical care services are provided are critical elements. If either is seen to be less than optimal, **a manageable epidemic could move toward catastrophe.**

Confronting a manageable epidemic and turning it into a catastrophe: that seems like a good description of everything that has happened in the COVID-19 crisis of 2020.

---

51 Glass et al. (2006).

52 See article herein entitled "How a Free Society Deals with Pandemics, According to Legendary Epidemiologist and Smallpox Eradicator Donald Henderson."

Thus did some of the most highly trained and experienced experts on epidemics warn with biting rhetoric against everything that the advocates of lockdown proposed. It was not even a real-world idea in the first place and showed no actual knowledge of viruses and disease mitigation. Again, the idea was born of a high-school science experiment using agent-based modelling techniques having nothing at all to do with real life, real science, or real medicine.

So the question becomes: how did the extreme view prevail?

*The New York Times* has the answer:[53]

> The [Bush] administration ultimately sided with the proponents of social distancing and shutdowns—though their victory was little noticed outside of public health circles. Their policy would become the basis for government planning and would be used extensively in simulations used to prepare for pandemics, and in a limited way in 2009 during an outbreak of the influenza called H1N1.[54] **Then the coronavirus came, and the plan was put to work across the country for the first time.**[55]

53 Lipton and Steinhauer (2020).

54 Navarro, J. Alexander, Katrin S. Kohl, Martin S. Cetron, and Howard Markel. 2016. "A Tale of Many Cities: A Contemporary Historical Study of the Implementation of School Closures during the 2009 pA(H1N1) Influenza Pandemic." *Journal of health politics, policy and law,* 41(3), 393–421.

55 Post-publication note: You can read the 2007 CDC paper here: https://www.cdc.gov/flu/pandemic-resources/pdf/community_mitigation-sm.pdf. It is arguable that this paper did not favor full lockdown. I've spoken to Rajeev Venkayya, MD, who regards the 2007 plan as more liberal, and assures me that they never envisioned this level of lockdown: "lockdowns and shelter-in-place were not part of the recommendations." To my mind, fleshing out the full relationship between this 2007 document and current policy requires a separate article.

*The Times* called one of the pro-lockdown researchers, Dr. Howard Markel, and asked what he thought of the lockdowns. His answer: he is glad that his work was used to "save lives" but added, "It is also horrifying." "We always knew this would be applied in worst-case scenarios," he said. "Even when you are working on dystopian concepts, you always hope it will never be used."

Ideas have consequences, as they say. Dream up an idea for a virus-controlling totalitarian society, one without an endgame and eschewing any experienced-based evidence that it would achieve the goal, and you might see it implemented someday. Lockdown might be the new orthodoxy but that doesn't make it medically sound or morally correct. At least now we know that many great doctors and scholars in 2006 did their best to stop this nightmare from unfolding. Their mighty paper should serve as a blueprint for dealing with the next pandemic.

## THE MODELS WERE WILDLY WRONG ABOUT REOPENING TOO

BY PHILLIP W. MAGNESS

July 23, 2020

Most of the United States entered into a tepid reopening from the COVID lockdowns in mid-May. Although the reopening process has advanced through an interminable succession of bureaucratic phases with most of the country remaining under varying degrees of restriction as of mid-July, the reopening process has remained under sustained criticism from the media and a segment of the epidemiology profession since the moment it started.

Back on May 24th the epidemiology team at Imperial College London (ICL) published a study that expanded on their now-notorious COVID-19 model.[56] Donald Trump and UK Prime Minister Boris Johnson both cited the apocalyptic projections of this report and its lead author Neil Ferguson back in March to justify their decisions to lock everything down.

The follow-up ICL paper from May attempted to model the effects of reopening in 5 US states: New York, Massachusetts, California, Washington, and Florida. In all five cases, the Imperial College team predicted an aggressive rebound of COVID-19 fatalities under even the most modest relaxation of stay-at-home policies and practices.

To illustrate this pattern, the ICL team presented three scenarios based on the expected change in human mobility in each state after the lifting of lockdown restrictions. The first scenario kept the lockdowns

---

56 Unwin, H Juliette T, Swapnil Mishra, Valeria C Bradley, Axel Gandy et al. 2020. "State-level tracking of COVID-19 in the United States." *Imperial College COVID-19 Response Team*, Report No. 23.

in place, assuming that mobility would remain constant at its severely reduced post-lockdown rate. Under the other two scenarios, the ICL team assumed a 20% and 40% increase of mobility corresponding with the reopening process.

In both of these reopening scenarios, the model depicted a catastrophic rebound of COVID-19 fatalities. As the ICL team itself put it, their model "illustrate[s] the potential consequences of increasing mobility across the general population: in almost all cases, after 8 weeks, a 40% return to baseline [mobility] leads to an epidemic larger than the current wave." Media reports at the time touted the study's dire warnings as reasons to stall the reopening process – even at its sluggish pace of recurring 2-week delays and extensions.[57]

More than 8 weeks have passed since the publication of the ICL team's warnings against reopening, meaning we can now see how their model performed.

As with other examples of ICL COVID modeling, their attempt to predict the effects of a US reopening can only be described as an embarrassing scientific failure.[58]

The image below shows the three modeled scenarios from May, as depicted in the ICL report for the five states under consideration. Note that even under the "constant mobility" scenario of remaining under lockdown, their model predicted an increase in COVID deaths for every state except New York, which had already peaked. Under the reopening scenarios where mobility increased 20% and 40% respectively from its lockdown state, all five states were predicted to surge into apocalyptic

57 Finucane, Martin. 2020. "Expert: A new study's dire picture of Mass. coronavirus future is a warning signal." *Boston Globe*, May 26.

58 See article herein entitled "SimCity-Style Modeling Flunks the Real-World Test."

territory by the middle of July. Under the 40% scenario, this even entailed upper boundaries of more than 4,000 deaths per day (the bands represent the 95% confidence interval). Massachusetts and New York, two of the hardest-hit states from the first wave back in March and April, would easily match or exceed their previous COVID-19 daily death records.

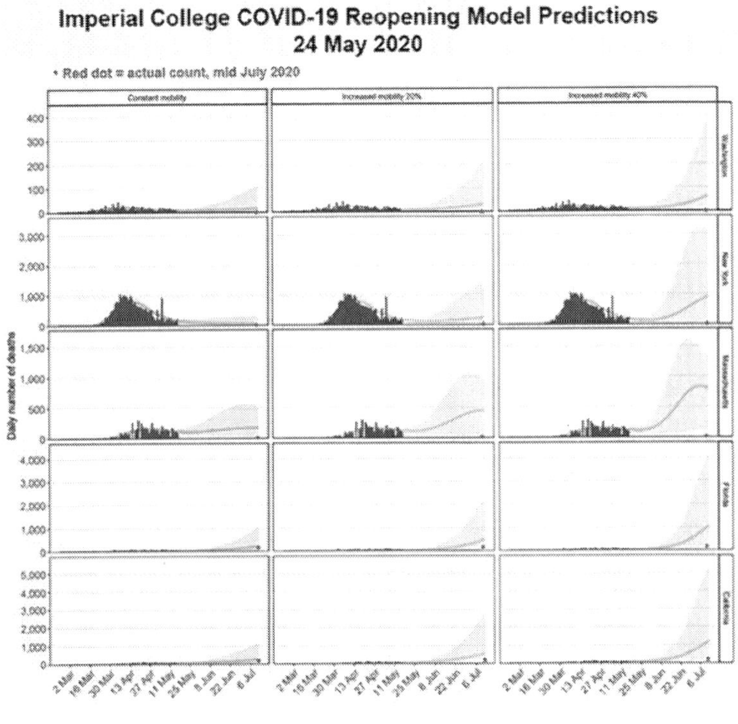


To see how these predictions held up, I indicated the daily death totals for each state for July 20th with a small red dot on the graphs above. As you can see, the actual totals are below the ICL model's predictions in every scenario. In Massachusetts, the current daily death totals are even falling below the lower boundary of the ICL model's projections for both its 20% and 40% mobility increase scenarios.

Coronavirus cases and deaths have spiked in two of the modeled states, Florida and California. As of the week of July 20th, both are averaging between roughly 100 and 150 deaths per day. Yet even with this "second wave" spike, Florida and California are only showing about one-tenth of the projected deaths that the Imperial College modelers predicted for this time back in May.

In New York, Washington, and Massachusetts, daily death counts have dropped to the low double-digits and remain a tiny fraction of the ICL predictions for mid-July.

Although all five states remain under COVID-19 restrictions of varying degrees, even partial reopening has increased mobility at levels that match or exceed the ICL's modeled scenarios. The main Google mobility indicators for Massachusetts are depicted below for reference, and show a clear upward trend since the time of the ICL predictions in mid-May.

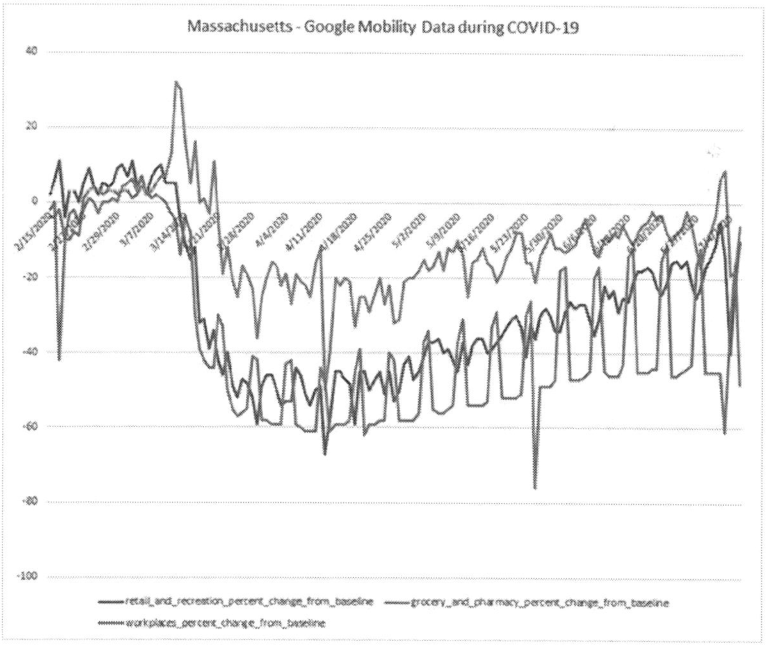

These patterns confirm that US mobility trends are increasing as lockdown restrictions are slowly lifted, and as society moves toward reopening. They therefore show that the ICL model correctly anticipated one effect of relaxing the lockdowns.

At the same time though, the ICL model severely overstated the projected mortality associated with reopening in all five states. Actual data do not map onto any of their scenarios, including the broadest of the three predictions for reopening. States that peaked back in March and April show no signs of a resurgence, let alone the predicted resurgence that would surpass the first wave. And states that are undergoing later surges are still well below the ICL team's predictions – so far below that they barely even register on the graphs.

As with other predictions from the ICL team, the May paper likely faltered due to a fundamental error in its underlying code. These flawed ICL models begin with an unproven assumption, namely that lockdowns are effective at combating the coronavirus. The models are therefore automatically calibrated to produce a sharp spike in deaths after the removal of lockdowns or any move toward reopening.

As we're now seeing in actual data however, that assumption is grossly exaggerated. As a result, the predictive ability of Imperial College's COVID epidemiology modeling amounts to little more than an exercise in statistical astrology.

## ANTI-LOCKDOWNERS WIN THE NUMBERS GAME THIS TIME. WHAT ABOUT THE NEXT TIME?

BY JOHN TAMNY

May 31, 2020

This article originally ran on RealClearMarkets

"If you are under 65, in reasonably good health and do not have a Vitamin D deficiency, you only have a tiny chance of dying from COVID-19. And if you are younger than 34, your chances of dying from the virus are so small as to almost be statistically undetectable."

Those are the words of my good friend Richard Rahn in his latest column for the *Washington Times*.[59]

Rahn very skillfully explodes the alarmism that has surrounded the spread of the new coronavirus. As of now, it's quite simply not much of a threat unless you're 85 or older, live "in a nursing home, [and] have serious health problems including a Vitamin D deficiency." Rahn thankfully notes that only "a tiny portion of the population is in such a condition."

So while Rahn's statistical breakdown of C-19 reads as great news, the view here is that there are dangers that come with turning debates about freedom into statistical battles. Rahn would likely agree.

To use an obvious example, Memphis is a city in zero tax rate, lightly regulated Tennessee. San Francisco is a city in heavily taxed, heavily regulated California. Yet a drive down Poplar in Memphis would reveal to the driver visually what's true empirically: Memphis's economy is

59 Rahn, Richard W. 2020. "'You are not going to die from COVID-19'." *The Washington Times*, May 25.

a small fraction of San Francisco's. Based on that, should Memphis and Tennessee adopt California's high-tax and high regulation way of doing things? After all, over half of the world's venture capital flows to the Golden State.

The Tennessee/California contrast is hopefully a reminder that freedom is its own virtue. The reality, as California's immense entrepreneurial wealth attests, is that talented people can still thrive to varying degrees despite all sorts of tax, regulatory and spending barriers. The goal should be less intrusive government regardless of outcome.

Applied to the virus, Rahn is plainly of the view that the lockdowns cruelly foisted on the electorate by local, state and national politicians have brought incalculable damage to the U.S. economy. No argument there. The lockdowns were and are a tragedy.

That they've been so disastrous speaks—at least partially—to why it's so dangerous to make the Covid argument a statistical one. To see why, consider what many well-meaning people will do with Rahn's excellent piece that yet again exposes the virus's microscopic lethality: they'll pass it around while concluding that it's time for the lockdowns to end. It all makes sense at first glance. But only at first glance. Please read on.

On second glance, it's easy to see just how dangerous such an approach is. That's the case simply because Covid-19 won't be the last virus to work its way around the world. Rest assured that when the next one rears its ugly (or largely benign) head, alarmist scientists, doctors, and self-styled experts will quickly have scared-of-their-own-shadow politicians lusting to "do something" to protect us from illness, and perhaps death.

Which is why those properly horrified by the lockdowns should re-focus the argument on freedom. Think about it.

If not about freedom, what happens if the expert conclusion about a future virus is that it's most lethal for those under 34? Implicit in all the statistical back-and-forth is that lockdowns might be justified then. Right? Young people are America's future and all that. Wrong.

Assuming a virus comes about that is said to favor old over young, then it's safe to say that the young will not need a law. Precisely because they're eager to live longer and healthier lives, they'll likely shelter-in-place on their own. What is it about avoiding getting sick or dying that requires force from politicians?

At the same time, there will be some young people for whom the threat of death means nothing. For those of the view that they're bulletproof in terms of health, some in the 34 and under range will continue living, working and traveling as though the virus is irrelevant. If so, great.

It's great because the assumptions and models created about most anything tend to not age very well. Lest readers forget, in the 1980s it was broadly thought that AIDS was an easily spreadable disease by contact. People avoided the afflicted like the plague. They no longer do because we now know that what the experts once thought to be true isn't.

With the coronavirus and future viruses, the same applies. Assuming one materializes that once again seems to hit 34 and under the hardest, the ideal is that some youthful types throw caution to the wind. Without their defiance, we can't really know the truth about why the virus spreads, and who is most endangered by it. Free people produce information.

It's all a reminder that lockdowns aren't just inexcusable because they destroy jobs, businesses and the human spirit. What takes away freedom is also anti-life. Lockdowns blind us as to what is best for us, and what will keep us safest when our safety is most imperiled.

In short, if we make the C-19 argument solely about numbers, we hand the very politicians who created so much economic misery the power to do so again. Let's not do that. But let's most crucially not allow lockdowns again because what crushes freedom also crushes the knowledge necessary to elongate life.

## THE FATAL CONCEIT OF COVID-19 EPIDEMIC MODELS

BY GREGORY VAN KIPNIS

June 10, 2020

With apologies to Friedrich Hayek, I find there is a fatal conceit amongst purveyors of epidemiological information that implies they know more than they can know when forecasting the outlook for a new infection. Of course, we have to do the best we can with limited information, but we should be humble in forecasting and reluctant to support politically inspired prescriptions of how society and the economy should be regulated in the face of uncertainty. We have to be very conservative because, more often than not, the first words out of a politician's mouth is "what's the worst case?" From that answer comes policy recommendations.

Be skeptical in the following sense. Long ago the great Austrian economist, Fritz Machlup, observed that in order to understand an economist (you can substitute the word "scientist") you need to know what interests he serves. For example, an economist from the chemical industry is unlikely to say anything negative about the outlook for that industry. So, it can be true for scientists due to the influence of funding sources they depend on.

### BASIC MODEL

Ever since the modelling work of Kermack and McKendrick in 1927, the mathematical description of how epidemics spread has grown in complexity, but the basic form remains the same. Below is described the five most basic equations that are extensions of their original work. It will be kept simple, but there is a major point to be made that is best understood if one has some understanding first of the equations used.

The key to validity is not the form of the equations, but the parameters to the equations. In early days those parameters need to be estimated with sparsely available data; therefore it is easy to reach conclusions that depend less on the certainty of facts than on the assumptions made. You get what you assume rather than getting what is justified by the facts to become known. Massage the input parameters and you get the outputs you desire. Recall the advice of Machlup.

The use of symbols is not to impress but to provide a sense of what we are talking about in a structured way. The first four equations are differential equations that describe the non-linear path of progression (in units of daily change). Specifically, they describe the propagation of an infection as it works its way through a population causing people to transition between four states starting with S, those that are susceptible, to E, those who are exposed, to I, those who are infected (also described as those who are infectious) and finally, R, those who have recovered. The states and the transitions from one to the next are pictured this way:

$S_t$ *(susceptible)* $\rightarrow E_t$ *(exposed)* $\rightarrow I_t$ *(infected/tious)* $\rightarrow R_t$ *(recovered)*

The changes (that's what ∂ means) in the number of people in each state per unit of time is described as follows:

1. $\delta S/\delta t = \mu N - \mu S - \beta SI/N$
2. $\delta E/\delta t = \beta SI/N - (\mu - \alpha)E$
3. $\delta I/\delta t = \alpha E - (\gamma - \mu)I$
4. $\delta R/\delta t = \gamma I - \mu R$
5. $R_0 = \alpha/(\mu + \alpha) \times \beta/(\mu + \gamma)$

The trajectory of the growth in deaths is derived indirectly by the difference between the infected (I) and the recovered (R).

The number of people in each group varies over time as people transition from group to group according to the probability of contact with someone who is infected, the probability the contact will result in an infection and the probability they will recover from the infection. The "Greek" symbols are expressions of the transition probabilities and have the following meaning:

$\beta$ = contact rate, i.e., the average number of contacts of a susceptible person per day, that is sufficient for disease transmission.

$\mu$ = mortality rate (% of group)

$\alpha$ = 1/average incubation period (as a % of a year)

$\gamma$ = 1/average infectious period (as a % of a year)

## THE R-NAUGHT BUGBOO

The 5th equation shows the calculation of a single number, the dreaded "reproduction number." Also referred to as R naught ($R_0$), it is the number of people that one person—that is, the first person to contract the disease—will infect at the onset of the disease.[60]

$R_0$ was made popular in the movie *Contagion*, so a large number of people have a passing familiarity with the concept. In the movie and in

60 Note that the reproduction number ($R_0$) is different from the number of recovered patients (R).

life there is a lot of anxiety over the correct value of $R_0$ because in the movie it would determine the fate of mankind in the absence of a cure.

In fact, $R_0$ is not directly measured. No one knows how many people were infected by the first infectious person. So, it has to be estimated as a point estimate, meaning it is a single number; that is derived from other numbers, which are themselves inimical to driving the entire hypothetical disease propagation. Though it is an initial condition which determines the behavior of the spread of an infection from the onset we will never directly measure it. It is very important that $R_0$ and its confidence interval are estimated as accurately as possible. However, several other equation parameters come into play, which they themselves are also estimated, and greatly affect the course of an epidemic.

An even bigger question, left unanswered in most academic papers you may read, is how did they come by this simple equation for $R_0$? Can it be observed directly or is it the byproduct of calculations solving the integrals for the differential equations 1-4, to determine the steady state outcome from initial assumed values of the parameters? This latter approach results in a so-called reduced-form derivation. Since, in the real world for a new disease, most of the parameters (the "Greeks") are unknown, a simulation can be run based on early tracking to estimate the parameters. Those estimates are improved upon over time as more data is obtained. Once the steady state outcome is calculated from the initial assumptions, a contact number, $R_0$, can be backward-derived. Many simplifying assumptions are made along the way.

In early days epidemiologists can try to estimate $R_0$ using contact tracing data obtained at the individual level. Who was the first to infect others is uncertain, so you search for the earliest patients who were diagnosed as infected. Their contacts are traced backward and each tested. $R_0$ is then computed by averaging the results for many diagnosed individuals. It is a crude approach.

The other approach is to obtain $R_0$ from cumulative data. This involves making assumptions based on ordinary differential equations that describe the dynamics at the population level of the number of people in each state without actually tracking specific individuals. It is very important to note that one method cannot be used to validate the other method. Mathematically, the relationship between the two calculations is considered complex and unknown.

From this point forward there is no need to further reference the differential equations 1-4 shown above. Instead, the focus will be on the calculation of the dreaded $R_0$. It is derived from four other values that are unknown at the onset of a new disease such as COVID-19. In fact, these values are not only difficult to estimate, but two of them are sure to change over time as the infected population adjusts to the reality of the infection. So whatever value is initially assumed for $R_0$ it is sure to change over time as well as with better data.

But here is the odd thing. The convention amongst epidemiologists is to leave $R_0$ unchanged; it is considered a "threshold" value. It is kept constant. They know that once over the "threshold" the reproduction rate will "evolve" but they call it something else. Furthermore, as will become clear from examples given below, very small errors of measurement of the inputs to the calculation of $R_0$ will have very large effects on the estimated "reproduction number" $R_0$.

It becomes obvious that any shortcomings in the objectivity and reporting of the early estimates of  can set off considerable fear and therefore likely result in wrong-headed personal and policy responses.

## EARLY ESTIMATES OF $R_0$

Health department spokesmen have given enormous emphasis in the press to the reproduction number $R_0$. It is treated with reverence and fear because, all other things being equal, if it is greater than 2 the infection can rapidly spread and lead to very high infection and death rates.

It seems like such a simple number with such high certainty attached to it. It is used in a way that it can be compared to the pass accuracy rate of a football quarterback. So-and-so has a 98% pass accuracy. But anyone who follows the game knows that you need to know a lot more if they are going to gain yardage on the field. You need to know if the intended receiver catches it, fumbles it, is bumped off, or it is intercepted. Just as it is true that you need to know more variables than just pass accuracy, it is equally the case for a disease. But it is even harder because a new disease is a one-time thing; it has no history. The rate of spread and lethality will not be known accurately until the end of the disease's propagation. As in football, there are defenses against an accurate passer, so is it true that many things will affect the course of a disease other than simply the $R_0$.

What have we been told about COVID-19's $R_0$?

- An early study for the CDC by a group of scientists at Los Alamos, using Chinese data, estimated $R_0$ at 5.7 with a confidence interval of 3.8 to 8.9.[61] A frighteningly high number.

---

61 Sanche, Steven, Yen Ting Lin, Chonggang Xu, Ethan Romero-Severson, Nick Hengartner, and Ruian Ke. 2020. "High Contagiousness and Rapid Spread of Severe Acute Respiratory Syndrome Coronavirus 2." *Emerging Infectious Diseases*, July, 26(7): 1470-1477.

- A later study based on data from Italy put the $R_0$ at 2.43 to 3.10.
- In another study a Harvard scientist suggested $R_0$ was in the 5 to 6 range.

For further perspective, calculations of $R_0$ for Rubella (German measles) was 6.4, for mononucleosis 2.2, for H3N2 (Hong Kong flu) 1.44 and for H2N2 (the Asian flu) 1.33.

Keep in mind that if $R_0$ is less than 1 there will not be an epidemic. It will die out quickly. If it is greater than 2 it is a very serious epidemic.

At this point serious work is no longer focused on estimation of the threshold value of $R_0$. That is considered yesterday's problem and it doesn't matter anymore, even if the estimate was wrong in the first place. Furthermore, the reproduction rate declines naturally anyway since the contact rate will decrease as the number of recovered cases increases thus reducing the number of people who can still be infected. Today the focus of politicians is to further reduce the reproduction rate by social engineering; that is, to force a reduction in contacts between the susceptible by social distancing.

Also, keep in mind that $R_0$ is a "statistical on average number." It can have about as much meaning as the statement that you will not drown crossing a river with an average depth of 3 feet. We all know how that can go wrong. At the individual level, the number of contacts vary widely based on age, region, occupation, etc. For example, for some spreaders (infectious people) the initial reproduction rate might be 12 and for others 0.

Even more important to the outcome of a disease is the recovery rate and the susceptibility rate. Those two factors are also not known until after the fact. Whether exposure will lead to an infection depends on the precautions taken on both sides of social intercourse. That is why people are encouraged to be extra careful in their sanitary habits because that likely will result in a significantly lower infection transmission rate.

As for the susceptibility rate, most epidemiologists assume that some portion is likely to have some sort of natural immunity. They can't be sure. They start with a zero assumption but as time goes on it is often discovered that exposure to some other disease has given some people an immunity or a decreased susceptibility to the new disease.

## HOMEMADE ESTIMATES OF $R_0$

OK, let's look at what goes into the estimation of $R_0$. From equation 5 (repeated below for convenience) we see that α, β, μ, and γ went into the calculation.

Recalling the reduced-form formula derived from the four partial derivative equations, and the parameter definitions:

$$R_0=\alpha/(\mu+\alpha)\ \times\beta/(\mu+\gamma)$$

$\beta$= contact rate, i.e., the average number of contacts of a susceptible person per day, that is sufficient for disease transmission.

$\mu$= mortality rate (% of group)

$\alpha$= 1/average incubation period (as a % of a year)

$\gamma$= 1/average infectious period (as a % of a year)

Notice there is a circularity in the calculation. At the get-go we need as an input the death or mortality rate ($\mu$). It is certainly a very

back upon past decisions is at times maddeningly inconclusive.[63]

So how do human beings solve problems? First, some NP-Hard problems are basically solvable using simple but powerful tools. While many of the decisions and challenges we face may technically be NP-Hard ("What degree program should I enter?"), we don't allow them to flourish in all of their intractable glory. While the definition of intelligence remains inconclusive, millions of years of evolution have resulted in the human mind coming "pre-loaded" with heuristics: we accumulate rules of thumb, put together past experiences to construct educated guesses, and we are born with the ability to conduct basic empirical analysis. All of these, further, are added to and honed with time and experience.

In short, human minds automatically jump over, cut through, and steer around uncountable solutions which are either obviously incorrect or don't meet other qualifications of our solution-seeking process, and focus only upon that set of solutions which appear to. And all along, time-preference, social, and cultural factors weigh into and influence the selection of our final choice. Moreover, success or failure of chosen heuristics influences both which ones and the order in which they are brought to bear on problems in the future, which has further influence on our problem-solving ability.

## WHAT'S THE POINT OF ALL THIS?

We have been watching, for months, as high-powered quantitative methods have been applied to interpret and predict the rapidly changing circumstances of a pandemic. And deeply embedded within that

---

63 Even when we tell ourselves we made the perfect choice at a perfect time or place, we are more likely engaging in harmless self-aggrandizement.

important number to know, but we won't know it until the epidemic has played out. The average infection period ($\gamma$) can be observed and averaged across patients if you know when the infected person became infected and how long it took for him to not be infectious. It means a lot of daily tests. The incubation period ($\alpha$) can also be measured if you know when they were exposed and when they came down with symptoms. Finally, there's the contact rate ($\beta$). That too is a guess. The contact rate is a number that estimates the average number of contacts a susceptible person experiences in a day that is sufficient for the transmission of the disease. It is not the total number of contacts one has but only that subset with those who are infectious and that those contacts must be serious enough that there could be transmission.

First, let's make some guesses at each parameter to get a feel for magnitudes and sensitivities. The values used in each of the cases described next are also recorded in the Table below.

## CASE #1

Assume the average incubation period is 10 days, then $\alpha$ is 0.1.

Assume a susceptible person comes into contact with 30 people in a day and 5% of them are infected and in close enough contact to cause transmission. Then the contact rate $\beta$ would be 1.5.

Further, assume the mortality (death) rate, $\mu$ is 1%.

Finally, assume the infection period is 5 days, then $\gamma$ is 0.2.

Solving for $R_0$ we get:

$$R_0 = 0.1/(0.01+0.1) \times 1.5/(0.01+0.2)$$
$$= 0.1/0.11 \times 1.5/0.21$$
$$= 0.909 \times 7.143$$
$$= 6.49$$

That value is similar to the early estimate based on Chinese data cited earlier.

## CASE #2

Evidence suggests the incubation period may be somewhat longer, e.g., 14 days. That causes $R_0$ to decrease slightly to 6.27.

## CASE #3

If the number of contacts "susceptibles" have with people who are infected, and where the contact is significant at 5%, drops to 20, then $R_0$ falls to 4.18.

The remaining 4 of the 7 cases show different combinations of assumptions of the parameters. Primarily the infection period is lengthened and the likelihood of an infection from a contact is reduced. By the 7th simulation, the initial estimate of $R_0$ drops to below 2.

***Simulated Calculations of $R_0$***

| Case | Incubation days | $\alpha$ | People contacted | % likely infected | $\beta$ | $\mu$ | Infection period | $\gamma$ | $R_0$ |
|---|---|---|---|---|---|---|---|---|---|
| #1 | 10 | 0.100 | 30 | 5.00% | 1.50 | 1.00% | 5 | 0.200 | 6.49 |
| #2 | 14 | 0.071 | 30 | 5.00% | 1.50 | 1.00% | 5 | 0.200 | 6.27 |
| #3 | 14 | 0.071 | 20 | 5.00% | 1.00 | 1.00% | 5 | 0.200 | 4.18 |
| #4 | 14 | 0.071 | 20 | 4.50% | 0.90 | 2.00% | 6 | 0.167 | 3.77 |
| #5 | 14 | 0.071 | 20 | 3.50% | 0.70 | 2.00% | 6 | 0.167 | 2.93 |
| #6 | 14 | 0.071 | 20 | 2.50% | 0.50 | 2.00% | 6 | 0.167 | 2.09 |
| #7 | 14 | 0.071 | 20 | 2.00% | 0.40 | 3.00% | 6 | 0.167 | 1.43 |

## CONCLUSION

The epidemiological world has published countless articles and studies warning against the tendency and ease with which one can overestimate $R_0$. We have fallen prey to this tendency once again. The Fatal

Conceit of bureaucrats in the service of politicians is that they imagine they know more than they actually need to know to design appropriate policy. They employ many scientists who struggle to maintain objectivity, but it is easy for those who control their budgets to pick and choose whose work they will support. Small errors of assumptions can produce large errors of policy.

When it is argued that it is "better to be safe than sorry," the response should be "how do you measure the value of 'safe?'" Number of sick, number of deaths, loss of freedom, loss to the economy? Is a loss of profits or GDP ever worth more than the loss of a life?

In war a general can ask for people to risk their lives for an objective. In peace time that ask can never be made.

The best answer would be to allow freedom of choice; that is, people should be granted the freedom to pursue personal preferences and arrangements. That freedom will result in manifold decisions. If left to the politician there will be only one decision, one that most assuredly will lead to a loss of personal and economic freedom.

## LIFE IS NP-HARD

BY PETER C. EARLE

July 29, 2020

On the 31st of July—just a few short days away—the six month anniversary of the WHO Declaration of a Global Health Emergency will arrive. And while there are many dates which could serve as the starting point for the start of the crisis, this one seems particularly appropriate: it is shortly thereafter that epidemiologists began plying the quantitative tools of their trade in force, and just after which the conversion from model outputs to policy schemes started to transpire.

We know now how dreadfully awry much of that planning went, not only in terms of harmless (if shockingingly wrong) predictions, but in real terms: lost lives, wealth, and opportunities. To the extent that epidemiological models attempt to predict or ascertain the infectious rate of a given pathogen, there is reason to believe that they can be helpful. But to the extent that those predictions, in turn, hinge upon decisions made by human beings—often by including a characteristic of an agent that replicates making choices—the effort is doomed to fail and, moreover, is an exercise in uncommendable audacity.

An overview of the taxonomy of problems underscores their incredible complexity, as well as the methods used to deal with them.

But first, I'm an economist; not a mathematician, computer scientist, or theoretical physicist. And tied to that, I have decided not to introduce such concepts of polynomial time, nondeterministic machines, and the like which are typically part of this discussion. I believe that, nevertheless, the deeply complicated nature of human thought and action in the face of uncertainty or impediments—and the futility of attempting to approximate those in models or simulations—will be made apparent.

## NP-COMPLETENESS

There are some problems which, on the surface, appear simple: putting a large number of irregularly shaped objects into a large box, for example. Obviously no two objects can occupy the same space at the same time. And while it may be easy to approach an optimal ordering of the irregular objects inside the box, it may be exceedingly difficult to determine the optimal structuring within the box. And further still, the difference between close-to-optimal ordering and actually optimal ordering may be small but nontrivial: for example, it may require unpacking every one of the irregular objects and starting over again.

It may be helpful to think of the solutions to a problem of this sort as a three-dimensional surface. If there are 500 irregular objects that we are required to place in the box – let's say that the requirement is to order all of the objects in a way that the box can be closed – and there are 50 undefined spaces within the box with 10 different possible orientations for each object, the problem would require (500 times 50 times 10) 250,000 bits to accurately represent every possible ordering within the box.

Now imagine that each of these possible orderings is evaluated by the amount of space that is left in the box, with a negative number representing a failure to be able to close the box and a positive number indicating a successful organization of objects within the box. Plotted in two dimensions, we would find a landscape: "sinkholes" or "valleys" in places, "hills" and "mountains" in others. Each "hill" represents a successful organization of objects within the box such that the box closes properly, and the optimal solution would be the highest "mountain" on our solution surface.

There are various algorithms which can be employed to solve such problems, and some are better than others.[62] Within this "solution surface" metaphor, such algorithms may start at a point, iteratively discard certain areas of the surface, and quickly bring us toward the area of the landscape that contains solutions; and ultimately, the optimal solution.

This is because this type of problem has an intrinsic structure to it. There is an ordering which may be simple or complex, but nevertheless exists; and given that it exists, it can be worked out and solved with enough computational power. We can not only find the best solution to the problem, but check and see that we have by running the problem over again.

## NP-HARDNESS

An NP-hard problem either has no such structure or the structure is so complicated as to be fundamentally impenetrable. In contrast to problems within the NP-Complete class, not only is such a problem difficult to solve, it is extremely difficult to determine if a chosen solution is the best one.

And the *coup de grace* of the NP-Hard class of problems? Proving that a problem is actually NP-Hard is itself an NP-Hard problem.

## COMPUTATIONAL COMPLEXITY IN EVERYDAY LIFE

Most of the time, and for good reason, the topic of computational complexity is relegated to masters and dissertation level courses in computer science (and sometimes physics). The problems they reference are vastly beyond putting irregularly shaped objects in a box: they're more along the lines of determining the existence of an optimal

---

62 The term "efficiency" in computational science is used to describe the time, memory, or number of steps taken to complete a computational task.

outcome to a game of generalized chess. Where the difficulty of finding a solution is concerned, they deal not with solutions that take hours or days but at times multiples of the theorized lifetime of the universe to compute. There is some debate over whether even quantum computers will be of use in solving the hardest of the NP-Hard problems.

But this class of difficult (often near impossible) problems to solve which are even more difficult (and perhaps effectively impossible) to check solutions to isn't consigned to scientific esoterica: human beings face them daily. Starting a new job, making decisions about saving or consumption, and a vast variety of other choices are, technically, NP-hard: even when binary decisions are involved, the number of considerations that make the perfect course of action is shrouded by uncertainty and changing situations, and that same array of conditions make looking back to determine if the correct option was selected an exercise in futility. Although we often give ourselves the benefit of the doubt, determining that in a past situation we picked the indisputably best alternative among what could be thousands of choices is probably not possible other than by force of sheer randomness.

Many NP-Hard problems, both in theory and in human life, involve optimization.

And I say "probably not possible," because as mentioned previously: proving that an issue falls within the category of NP-Hard is itself NP-Hard. I can't prove it, and even if I could it would be impracticable for me or anyone else to substantiate.

## IF SO MUCH IS UNSOLVABLE, HOW DO WE SOLVE ANYTHING?

If this framing sounds nihilistic, it isn't meant to; nor is the epistemological concept itself. Few would be surprised to learn that there are some questions for which there will never be clear answers, or that looking environment are a variety of social science issues. But despite sometimes acknowledging the challenges of boiling down the actions of hundreds of millions or billions of people to agents in an agent-based model or nodes and arcs in a network model, that method of informing policy seems to be continuing unabated.

Inside the mind of every individual, scores of NP-Hard problems are being worked out: some so quickly as to be instantaneous, and others in a stepwise fashion of days, years, or decades. In the aggregate, deciphering the ways in which enormous masses of individuals will move or act is, similarly, an NP-Hard problem. The outcome of the collisions of individual responses to NP-Hard problems (and, to be sure, all of the other problems in other categories that people face) is utterly and wholly unpredictable; as intractable in the aggregate as in each of hundreds of millions or billions of minds.

Life is NP-Hard, and attempting to express that mentation in a few lines of code is imprudent, yet in and of itself probably harmless. But bringing those projected outcomes to politicians, who have neither the inclination to be skeptical or incentives to act cautiously, is dangerous.

## THE MODELERS THOUGHT OF EVERYTHING EXCEPT REALITY

BY AIER STAFF

June 14, 2020

As a site focused on economics, AIER would rather have stayed away from commentary on diseases and their mitigation. In normal times, we would have.

The archives of AIER dating back to 1933 show that we had no comments on the polio epidemic (1948-1951), the Asian Flu (1957-59), the Hong Kong flu (1968-69), the Avian bird flu (2006), or the Swine flu pandemic of 2009, which was a strain most like 1918 and therefore, one might suppose, would have caused panic but did not.

We had nothing to say because disease mitigation is a job for medical professionals, not economists and certainly not politicians.

The problem is that this time, the disease mitigators (some of them, the ones in power and with the ear of politicians) didn't stay out of economics. Indeed, their plans for mitigation trampled all over commerce, life, and the freedoms that are necessary to make it function. For a few months in 2020, the presumptuous model-building disease mitigators became central planners, overriding the wisdom of not only medical professionals but also economists, philosophers, political scientists, historians, and everyone else including legislatures and voters.

Our first piece on the topic ran January 27.[64] The focus was on the quarantine power and the argument was simple: because people are not ridiculous and know how to deal with disease in consultation with medical professionals, this state power should not be deployed. At the

---

64 Tucker, Jeffrey A. 2020. "Must Government Save Us from the Coronavirus?" *American Institute for Economic Research*, January 27.

time, people said we were being alarmist even for saying this. Nothing like this could ever happen in the U.S. because we have a Constitution and courts and a tradition of trusting the people.

It turns out, of course, that we underestimated the threat of coercion. It wasn't just about quarantining the sick. It was about putting the whole of the country (but for a few governors who heroically resisted) under lockdown. This brought about economic collapse (and increasingly social and cultural collapse too). We chronicled the disaster in real time on this site, which became an essential go-to source for factual information and rational analysis—in contrast to the mainstream media which was pushing for panic and lockdown.

On April 2, we published our first set of commentaries: *Coronavirus and Economic Crisis*, edited by Peter C. Earle.[65] Amazon would not permit the Kindle edition to go live. They have admitted to us that they "incorrectly blocked" the book. There is no going back but it remains a reality: AIER's influence was blocked when it was most needed. It's the fourth time in our history we've been censored.

The following book you recently submitted have been reviewed and were successfully passed:

Coronavirus and Economic Crisis by Earle, Peter (AUTHOR) (ID: 34713542)

We incorrectly blocked your book and apologize for the inconvenience this caused.

The book will soon be published on Amazon. Please allow up to 48 hours for the book to become available in the Amazon Store.

Those were censorious times. It is however available now.

Much of the commentary focused on the absurd failures of the models being used by a handful of statisticians and epidemiologists. They predicted as many as 2.3 million deaths in the United States (the

65 Earle, Peter C. 2020. *Coronavirus and Economic Crisis. American Institute for Economic Research:* EBook.

*New York Times* went one better and predicted 8.25 million deaths) if government didn't crack down and shutter nonessential business, and lock hospitals down to become COVID-only zones.

Economists know something about the incredible failure of forecasting models. They have been deployed often in the postwar period. They came under heavy fire from economists of the Austrian and classical schools. They don't grapple with certain facts of reality: second and third tier responses to policies, unpredictabilities of human choice, and the uncertainties of the future. There are too many variables operating in a complex system like a socio-economic order for any mechanistic model to capture them all, especially when dealing with an unknown and unknowable future.

The same forecasting failures afflicted the models that panicked politicians into locking down. They are too aggregated. They don't consider population diversity and how novel viruses affect different groups in different ways. They presume that planners can know things that they cannot know, such as disease severity in the midst of an epidemic. Slogans like "flatten the curve" massively oversimplify social processes and human choices, and presume to know far too much about cause and effect.

It turned out of course that the models were horribly wrong, not only about the large death numbers but also about hospital capacity, unseen costs, economic effects, and even the demographics of the affected population. Remarkably, none of the models even considered the impact of the virus on long-term care facilities, and hence contributed to gross neglect of the population that should have received the bulk of the focus.

*The Wall Street Journal* sums up the blizzard of data rather sharply:[66]

> About 80% of Americans who have died of Covid-19 are older than 65, and the median age is 80. A review by Stanford medical professor John Ioannidis last month found that individuals under age 65 accounted for 4.8% to 9.3% of all Covid-19 deaths in 10 European countries and 7.8% to 23.9% in 12 U.S. locations.
>
> For most people under the age of 65, the study found, the risk of dying from Covid-19 isn't much higher than from getting in a car accident driving to work. In California and Florida, the fatality risk for the under-65 crowd is about equal to driving 16 to 17 miles per day. While higher in hot spots like New York (668 miles) and New Jersey (572 miles), the death risk is still lower than the public perceives.

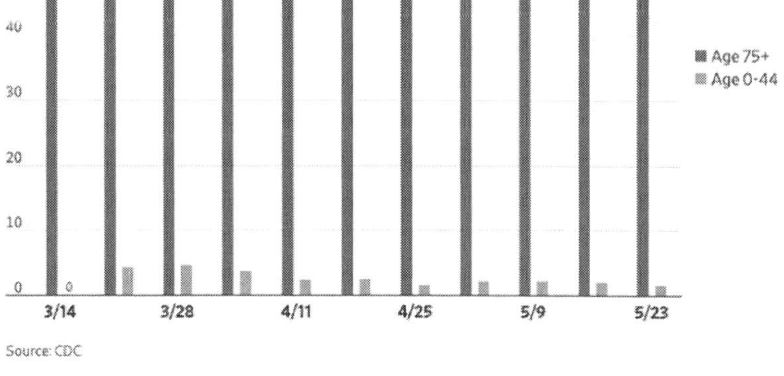


66 WSJ Editorial Board. 2020. "The Covid Age Penalty." *The Wall Street Journal*, June 12.

Future historians will be astonished to ruminate about what we did here. We shut down schools, sports, theaters, bars, restaurants, and churches—government ignored the rule of law and put individual rights on hold—but it is more than obvious now that this was all a huge distraction. The focus should have been on the aged with underlying conditions living in nursing homes.

The models nowhere included what ended up being our reality, even though that reality was upon us as early as February when people in nursing homes began to die in Washington State. We should have seen it long before the lockdowns began.

Now the modelers in the epidemiological profession need to learn what the economists figured out long ago. Human life is too complex to be accurately modeled, much less predicted. This certainly pertains to a novel virus.

Economics in the 18th and 19th centuries focused on logic and principles. Economists sought to discern laws that operate in the material world, how incentives affect human choice, where wealth comes from, how production works, the function of prices, and they sought to introduce to the human mind accurate and realistic theories of the relationship between the material world and the human experience. Over the centuries, economics became a beautiful science.

In the 20th century, that way of understanding economics came under scrutiny as a new generation of thinkers began to imagine a better way. John Maynard Keynes in the 1930s famously rejected classical theorems but the problems had begun much earlier and lasted much longer. Eventually, economics was saddled with a thing called modeling—a technical approach that eschewed real-world data and experience for computer simulations.

The American Institute for Economic Research has been fighting against this way for its entire history. Along with our work has been some of the best economic minds of the 20th century: Ludwig von Mises, F.A. Hayek, Benjamin Anderson, Joseph Schumpeter, and so on.

It seems like epidemiology similarly took a turn for the worse around 2006, when agent-based modeling strategies displaced the accumulated wisdom of the ages as summed up by Donald Henderson in this beautiful piece we republished.[67]

It is not implausible to think that we can all get smart again about modeling and viruses. Consider the words of South Dakota Governor Kristi Noem. She never locked down. She resisted.[68]

> So this brings me to the question of modeling. While modeling certainly has a place, models have two major shortcomings. No model can actually predict the future. Especially when it is based on data that is incomplete. And no model is capable of replacing human freedom as the best path to responding to life's risks, including this virus.
>
> That is why central planning of the economy has failed every time the government has tried it. In South Dakota, we saw modeling as a tool, and we used it to be prepared for a worst case scenario. I thank God that the worst case hasn't happened. But we were ready, and we are still ready, if it does.
>
> But there is no model that can take into consideration all of

---

67 See articles herein entitled "The 2006 Origins of the Lockdown Idea" and "How a Free Society Deals with Pandemics, According to Legendary Epidemiologist and Smallpox Eradicator Donald Henderson."

68 Noem, Kristi (@govkristinoem). 2020. "About modeling…" *Twitter*, June 10, 2020. https://twitter.com/govkristinoem/status/1270751326373208064

> the factors that make real life work. A blind reliance on insufficient modeling has led some politicians to institute disastrous lockdowns, that have not only jeopardized their people's health, and their welfare, but also created conditions for a financial catastrophe, that will cause untold burdens and costs on their people for generations.

A powerful June 5, 2020, editorial in the *Journal of the American Medical Association* makes the core point:[69]

> Both modelers and public health policy makers should recognize that COVID-19 is not a unitary epidemic; in the US and other countries, it likely consists of multiple, contemporaneous, and intertwined suboutbreaks prominently including those in LTC settings. Distinguishing the rates and pattern of disease occurring in the general population from those in LTC facilities is both feasible and critical to control of infection in these high-risk settings. Creating separate models that reflect how COVID-19 has affected these different populations could provide more accurate evidence to guide mitigation efforts in the community and in LTC facilities, and could be helpful to better understand and reduce the morbidity and mortality this infection has caused among the most frail and vulnerable individuals.

---

69 Pillemer, Karl, Lakshminarayana Subramanian, and Nathaniel Hupert. 2020. "The Importance of Long-term Care Populations in Models of COVID-19." *JAMA*, 324(1): 25-26.

We doubt the ability to create better models, however. Viruses do not behave in real life as they do in World of Warcraft and Hollywood movies.[70] People are not automatons. They are choosing minds capable of intelligent adaptation to new realities, even pandemics. Instead we absolutely must recapture the wisdom of the past if we are going to deal intelligently with viruses in the future.

We cannot centrally plan an economy. Computers are no help. We cannot centrally plan a response to a new virus. Computers are of no help. For the sake of health, prosperity, human rights, and liberty, leave disease mitigation to the professionals and get it out of the hands of modelers and the politicians they intimidate into implementing their plans.

---

70 See article herein entitled, "World of Warcraft's Corrupted Blood Outbreak is Not a Model for COVID-19."

# MISUSE OF STATISTICS

## THE COLUMBIA-NYT MODEL CAN'T BE RIGHT

BY ROBERT E. WRIGHT

March 21, 2020

*The New York Times* has headlined an article and several interactive maps, based on research conducted by researchers at Columbia University.[71] The maps purportedly show the spread of COVID-19 infections over the next few months across the continental United States by county under three scenarios: no control measures, some control measures, and severe control measures.

It's riveting, engaging, alarming.

Also, it cannot be correct.

Under the "no transmission reduction" scenario the infection rate for almost every county in the entire United States is predicted to exceed 65 percent and in many places is predicted to exceed 90 percent. Such high rates would be unprecedented in epidemiological history, underdeveloped as that field is, and exceed the CDC's own worst-case scenario.[72]

True, the virus is "novel" but infection rates naturally cannot exceed about 65 percent. To see why, consider that the number of new infections on a given day is determined by those infected on the previous day times their average number of contacts with *uninfected*

---

71 Glanz, James, Lauren Leatherby, Matthew Bloch, Mitch Smith, Larry Buchanan et al. 2020. "Coronavirus Could Overwhelm U.S. Without Urgent Action, Estimates Say." *The New York Times,* March 20.

72 Webb, James L.A. 2015. "The historical epidemiology of global disease challenges." *The Lancet* January 24; Danner, Chas. 2020. "CDC's Worst-Case Coronavirus Model: 214 Million Infected, 1.7 Million Dead." *New York Magazine*, March 13.

persons (1 – proportion infected) times the probability of transmission per contact.

Controls like social distancing, hand washing, shuttering businesses and such are meant to reduce the average number of contacts and the probability of transmission per contact.

But note that the number of uninfected persons declines as the number of infected increases, naturally slowing the spread of the infection. Think of it as the law of diminishing returns applied to biology. The proper models are logistic, not exponential. In other words, when plotted they look like S curves, not moonshots. If this doesn't make sense to you, check out this video.[73]

Also, many of the county-level predictions look dubious. I will concentrate my critique on South Dakota, where I have lived since 2009. While I have not set foot in every county in the state, hunting, fishing, traveling, and research (for *Little Business on the Prairie*) has given me a good feel for most of it.[74]

I cannot fathom an approximate 60% infection rate for Miner and Sanborn counties by 1 May with no controls or by 10 June with some controls. The roughly 30% predicted by 1 August with severe controls also seems outlandish, even though most of the denizens of those counties are ranchers and farmers of a politically conservative bent not likely to allow Washington, or even Pierre (South Dakota's capital), to impose severe controls on them.

Most South Dakotans simply live too far apart. Sure, they congregate in churches and local bars and restaurants, like *Animal* in Canova

---

73 3Blue1Brown. 2020. "Exponential growth and epidemics." *YouTube*, March 8.

74 Wright, Robert E. 2015. *Little Business on the Prairie: Entrepreneurship, Prosperity, and Challenge in South Dakota.* Sioux Falls, South Dakota.

(Miner Co.), but not often or in large numbers, especially during planting and calving season. Normally, they travel to Sioux Falls or Rapid City about once a month to stock up but they likely have already stocked up on essentials like everyone else. Those who didn't prepare have neighbors or relatives who will help them out and there is plenty of fat and protein around for everybody: cattle, sheep, hogs, chickens, fish, and, in a pinch even if they are out of season, deer and pheasants. Plenty of switchgrass and corn cobs for the bathroom duties too.

Most can make their own alcohol if need be. I don't know if they can make their own smoke too and both interest rates and the stock market are (somehow) down, but Hank Williams, Jr. pretty much has the situation pegged in his song "Country Boy Can Survive."[75]

Rural South Dakotans are friendly enough, if you aren't trespassing on their land, but most don't want to shake your hand even in normal times and anyway are probably wearing a glove covered with snow, placenta, or entrails, depending on the season.

I am only partly in jest but the notion that 69% of the residents of rural McCook County will be infected while only 40% of the residents of Minnehaha, home of the much more densely populated Sioux Falls, will be infected seems far-fetched at best. I believe that the death rates will be higher in rural counties due to their gerontological age structure but that too suggests that infection rates will be lower.

West River (that means west of the Missouri for the coastal elites reading this) remains John Birch Society country.[76] The Colum-

---

75 Hank Williams, Jr. 2011. "Hank Williams, Jr. - "A Country Boy Can Survive" (Official Music Video)." *YouTube*, August 2.

76 Abourezk, James G. 1898. "Advise & Dissent: Memoirs of South Dakota and the U.S. Senate." Lawrence Hill Books: USA. At p. 11.

bia-*Times* model reveals a similarly bizarre pattern there, with Rapid City, the state's second biggest city, predicted to have a lower rate of infection than rural Lyman, and not much higher rates than almost unpopulated counties in the Black Hills. The biggest restaurant in Deerfield Reservoir (Pennington County) seats about 20 tops and will be lucky to have more than 5 patrons at one time this year, no matter what official controls are in place. In case your parents never took you on a 40-hour car trip to Mount Rushmore, this is what a lot of the West River part of the state looks like.[77] Those are dinosaur (fossil) hunting grounds, not avant-garde buildings, and hardly breeding grounds for a pandemic.

Another oddity is that the state's Indian Reservations are predicted to come through the pandemic relatively unscathed. Unfortunately, the researchers coded their stuff in an arcane programming language so it is difficult to observe exactly what they did but apparently the lack of roads on Reservations is predicted to save them. There is something to that but the lack of cars also means that hitchhiking is still commonly practiced although it is just as illegal and frowned upon on Reservations as elsewhere.[78] Plus there are some cultural beliefs and practices that might increase infection rates along with, you know, the grinding poverty and inept Indian Health Services.[79]

Of course no model can include everything; like the communal

77 NPS. 2020. "Land of Stone and Light." *National Park Service.*

78 See Ian Frazier's *On the Rez.*

79 Wikipedia. 2020. "List of South Dakota locations by per capita income." *Wikipedia*, April 4; Weaver, Christopher, Dan Frosch, and Lisa Schwartz. 2019. "The U.S. Gave Troubled Doctors a Second Chance. Patients Paid the Price." *The Wall Street Journal*, November 22.

living style of South Dakota's Hutterites, in which all members of each colony are likely to get infected, but only if any of them do. But the Columbia-*Times* model seems a lot like the simple money multiplier model in macroeconomics principles textbooks, i.e., one divided by the reserve requirement. It misses a lot of natural brakes to disease spread (deposit expansion) and hence overestimates, by a lot.

It also seems disingenuous to claim such precision based on 14 confirmed cases of COVID-19 in the state to date, out of 663 negative tests of those considered at-risk.[80] I could use that data and a simple model to concoct three Alfred E. Neuman-style "What Me Worry" scenarios.[81] But I won't because the independent AIER has more integrity than the *New York Times*, a commercial enterprise more dependent on attracting eyeballs than serving the public interest.[82]

This is just one state. A similar critique could be made of every spot on the map. Most of the disease-forecasting models hitting the headlines these days are based on applying dubious exponentials on vast numbers of unknowns, while the public-relations spin weaves the appearance of certainty that is unsustainable given existing knowns.[83]

---

80 Welte, Dean. 2020. "South Dakota reports 3 new cases of COVID-19, state total now 14." *KTIV*, March 19.

81 Wikipedia. 2020. "Alfred E. Neuman." *Wikipedia*, July 1.

82 Wright, Robert E. 2019. "What Economic News Can You Trust?" *American Institute for Economic Research*, September 2.

83 Resnick, Brian. 2020. "The 9 most important unanswered questions about Covid-19." *Vox*, March 20.

## AN EGREGIOUS STATISTICAL HORROR STORY

BY GEORGE GILDER

April 24, 2020

This piece originally ran at RealClearMarkets

With the latest reports of plummeting death rates from all causes, this crisis is over. The pandemic of doom erupted as a panic of politicians and is now a comedy of MASH-minded medical administrators and stooges, covering their "ifs," "ands," and "butts" with ever more morbid and distorted statistics.

The crisis now will hit the politicians and political Doctor Faucis who gullibly accepted and trumpeted what statistician William Briggs calls "the most colossal and costly blown forecast of all time."[84]

An egregious statistical horror story of millions of projected deaths, suffused with incense and lugubrious accents from Imperial College of London to Harvard School of Public Health, prompted the political elites to impose a vandalistic lockdown on the economy. It would have been an outrage even if the assumptions were not wildly astronomically wrong.

Flattening the curve was always a fool's errand that widened the damage.

President Trump had better take notice. He will soon own this gigantic botch of policy and leadership. No one will notice that his opponents urged even more panicky blunders.

The latest figures on overall death rates from all causes show no

84 Briggs, William M. 2020. "Coronavirus Update X: Juicing The Numbers, Prolonging The Pain." *William M. Briggs*, April 21.

increase at all. Deaths are lower than in 2019, 2018, 2017 and 2015, slightly higher than in 2016. Any upward bias is imparted by population growth.

Now writing a book on the crisis with bestselling author Jay Richards, Briggs concludes: "Since pneumonia deaths are up, yet all deaths are down, it must mean people are being recorded as dying from other things at smaller rates than usual." Deaths from other causes are simply being ascribed to the coronavirus.

As usual every year, deaths began trending downward in January. It's an annual pattern. Look it up. Since the lockdown began in mid-March, the politicians cannot claim that their policies had anything to do with the declining death rate.

A global study published in Israel by Professor Isaac Ben-Israel, chairman of the Israeli Space Agency and Council on Research and Development, shows that "the spread of the coronavirus declines to almost zero after 70 days—no matter where it strikes, and no matter what measures governments impose to try to thwart it."[85]

In fact, by impeding herd immunity, particularly among students and other non-susceptible young people, the lockdown in the U.S. has prolonged and exacerbated the medical problem. As Briggs concludes, "People need to get out into virus-killing sunshine and germicidal air."

This flu, like all previous viral flus, will give way only to herd immunity, whether through natural propagation of an extremely infectious pathogen, or through the success of one of the hundreds of vaccine projects.

No evidence indicates that this flu was exceptionally dangerous. On

---

85 Ben-Israel, Isaac. 2020. "The end of exponential growth: The decline in the spread of coronavirus." *The Times of Israel*, April 19.

March 20th, the French published a major controlled study that shows no excess mortality at all from coronavirus compared to other flus. SARS and MERS were both much more lethal and did not occasion what Briggs' reader "Uncle Dave" described as "taking a hammer and sickle to the economy."

We now know that the crisis was a comedy of errors. The Chinese let it get going in the raw bat markets of Wuhan. But together with the Koreans, the Chinese dithered and demurred and allowed six weeks of rampant propagation to create herd immunity before they began locking everyone up. Therefore, the Chinese and Koreans were among the first to recover.

The Italians scared everybody with their haphazard health system and smoking fogies. Crammed together in subways and tenements, the New Yorkers registered a brief blip of extreme cases. Intubations and ventilators turned out not to help.[86] This sowed fear and frustration among medical personnel slow to see that the problem was impaired hemoglobin in the blood rather than lung damage.

The New York media piled on with panic, with bogus reports of rising deaths. "Coronavirus deaths" soared by assuming that people dying with the virus were dying from it and then by ascribing to the coronavirus other deaths among people with symptoms of pulmonary distress, even without being tested.

Now jacking up the case rate will be further pointless testing. As Briggs points out,

Fauci is calling for 'tripling' of testing, which can only boost these dailies [case totals]. And make it seem like there's a genuine increase

86 80 percent died.

occurring. Oh my! The daily reported cases are up! It must mean the disease is spreading!

> No. It could also mean, and probably does given all the other evidence we now have from sampling, that the disease was already there, and we just now have measured it.

The death rate rises with further reclassification of pneumonia and other pulmonary deaths. When we reach herd immunity, and nearly everyone has the antigen, nearly all deaths can be chalked up to COVID-19. Hey, it will be *Quod Erat Demonstrandum* for the panic mongers.

In a fascinating open letter to German Prime Minister Angela Merkel, epidemiologist Mihai Grigoriu concludes that with the French study, corroborated by findings from a Stanford antibody seroprevalence study in Santa Clara county, "the case for extreme measures collapses like a house of cards." Grigoriu says that since the virus has already spread widely in the general population, efforts to stop further spread are both futile and destructive.

So let's stop pretending that our policies have been rational and need to be phased out, as if they once had a purpose. They should be reversed summarily and acknowledged to be a mistake, perpetrated by statisticians with erroneous computer models.

Perhaps then we can learn from this experience with the flaws of expertise not to shut down the economy again for the totally bogus "crisis" of climate change.

## MOST PLACES ARE NOT NEW YORK: A LOOK THROUGH THE COVID-19 DATA

BY JAMES L. CATON

May 14, 2020

Dr. Erickson:

> A state like New York... the state of New York, an entire state, has 19.4 million. In... New York City they are really close together. Where I live, in Kern County, we have 900,000 people, it's one of the biggest counties in California. Everyone is spread out. We drive cars. We don't ride the subway... If they said, doctor, how would you open up New York and how would you open up California. Would you have a same or a different strategy?[87]

Dr. Wittkowski:

> ...[I]f it's closely populated like New York, you can get very high spikes. In a country that is not very closely populated you would never have such a high spike because it takes more time for the virus to travel from one place to the next. So I think there is no reason anywhere in the United States to say "we need to continue with this second prohibition."[88]

As of writing today, we have observed for two consecutive days U.S. death tolls that are at their lowest since March.[89] Not to raise our

87 @max.eastman. 2020. "Dr. Erickson Interviewing Dr. Wittkowski - May 2020." *lbry.tv*, May 13.

88 Ibid.

89 Worldometer. 2020. "United States Coronavirus Cases." *Worldometer*, May 14.

hopes, Dr. Anthony Fauci has advised that we should expect to be homeschooling our children in the fall.[90] Are conditions so bad that we will not be past the peak of the curve by the end of the month? And even if we are not, allowing the spread to occur among younger students has been precisely the opposite approach than taken by Germany and Sweden, countries that have fared relatively well over the last two months.[91] So which is it? Are we in a year-long crisis where even spread among children is dangerous, or have we reached a point where voluntary precautions are enough to allow a return to normalcy?

Here at AIER we have documented that most of the early models over predicted the number of deaths by a magnitude of greater than 10.[92] As Yogi Bera once said, "It's tough to make predictions, especially about the future." In this spirit, a recent article in *The Spectator* makes the plea that "It is data, not modeling that we need now."[93] We have plenty of data. It's just a matter of making good use of that data.

Following *The Spectator*'s suggestion, I reviewed county level COVID-19 data from Johns Hopkins, perhaps shedding light on

---

90 Hall, Colby. 2020. "You'll Still Be Homeschooling Your Kids This Fall, Dr. Fauci Says." *BestLife*, May 12.

91 Safi, Marlo. 2020. "Germany To Begin Opening Schools And Shops But Ban Public Gatherings Until August 31." *Daily Caller*, April 15; Romano, Andrew. 2020. "Should Americans look to Sweden or Germany as a model for combating coronavirus?" *Yahoo News*, May 12.

92 Luther, William J. 2020. "More Sensational Reporting on COVID-19 Estimates." *American Institute for Economic Research*, March 27; Magness, Phillip W. 2020. "Imperial College Model Applied to Sweden Yields Preposterous Results." *American Institute for Economic Research*, April 30; Magness, Phillip W. 2020. "How Wrong Were the Models and Why?" *American Institute for Economic Research*, April 30.

93 Ridley, Matt. 2020. "We know everything – and nothing – about Covid." *The Spectator*, May 9.

conflicting opinions of Dr. Fauci, representing the disposition of many providing advice to policymakers, on one hand, and Nobel Laureate Michael Levitt, Professor Johan Giesecke, Dr. Knut Wittkowski and Dr. David Katz who suggest that we allow the virus to spread while sheltering the vulnerable.[94]

Nearly two weeks have passed since the start of reopening of states across the U.S.; COVID-19 continues to spread, but there are reasons to be hopeful. Most of the United States has been able to avoid the overload of local medical systems experienced in New York and other Northeastern states where the virus has spread. New York City has been the epitome of conditions to avoid in this regard.

The virus arrived early in New York and had considerable time to spread across the population. Unaccustomed to pandemic and guided by political leadership, individuals were slow to adjust their daily behavior.[95] In most places, the situation might not have turned sour so quickly, but heavy use of public transit and the nature of living within America's most densely populated city promoted a fast spread. Before the end of April, researchers estimated that greater than 20% of New Yorkers had contracted the coronavirus, as compared to around 5% of

---

94 Data.world. 2020. "COVID-19 Activity Dataset by Coronavirus (COVID-19) Data Hub." *Data.world*, March; UnHerd. 2020. "Nobel prize winning scientist Prof Michael Levitt: lockdown is a 'huge mistake.'" *YouTube*, May 2; UnHerd. 2020. "Why lockdowns are the wrong policy - Swedish expert Prof. Johan Giesecke.'" *YouTube*, April 17; Stringham, Edward Peter. 2020. "Stand Up for Your Rights, says Bio-Statistician Knut M. Wittkowski." *American Institute for Economic Research*, April 6; Stringham, Edward Peter. 2020. "'Don't Destroy People's Lives and Livelihoods,' says Dr. David L. Katz." *American Institute for Economic Research*, April 29.

95 Goodman, J. David. 2020. "How Delays and Unheeded Warnings Hindered New York's Virus Fight." *The New York Times*, April 8.

Californians in Los Angeles and Santa Clara Counties.[96]

Thankfully, we have not yet seen anything comparable to the spread in New York. Most American cities are not comparable to New York City. And much of the U.S. is rural or at least not very densely populated. With less interactions per person in these areas, the rate of spread tends to be much lower. Thus, many counties in the middle of the U.S. have not recorded even a single death involving COVID-19 as of May 12, the most recent date for which Johns Hopkins provides data.

*While there have been other local spreads*, such as those in southwestern Georgia and across Louisiana, overall the rate of spread has been slow. Deaths from COVID-19 as a portion of the population in Georgia's most populous counties has been limited in comparison to some rural southwest counties in the state. These are the exceptions.

In many areas across the U.S., residents have had time to internalize norms of social distancing and actively maintain standards of hygiene that limit the chance of contracting the virus. Those who are vulnerable have had more time to develop strategies to protect themselves. The increase in cases in many of the areas where spread occurred relatively slowly has not been accompanied by an increase in the level of fatalities comparable to the northeast. Probably another month or more will need to pass before one can express confident judgment. Still, this is an encouraging sign that precautions to protect the vulnerable have been effective.

## COMPARING THE EVOLUTION OF SPREAD

Below I have included graphs of counties by state, comparing the

---

96 Goodman, J. David, and Michael Rothfeld. 2020. "1 in 5 New Yorkers May Have Had Covid-19, Antibody Tests Suggest." *The New York Times*, April 23.

deaths from COVID-19 within each county as a proportion of county population. It is helpful to judge the spread according to the slope of the curves. The grey lines indicate a doubling of deaths every 2, 3, or 5 days from the first day that at least 0.0001 percent of the population had died from COVID-19. Since the data is normalized by population, it is also fair to compare curve levels.

Whether or not you are concerned about overcounting, as indicated by this CDC measure, it is the rate of spread that concerns us in regard to the capacity of the medical system.[97] A persistent doubling of deaths, say, every two days or less indicates a system that is being incapacitated by the coronavirus. Most counties have experienced a doubling of deaths from coronavirus about every five days or longer. Spread in nearly every region outside of the Northeast has been relatively tame.

Compared to other states, New York and neighboring states experienced high death rates in the earliest days of the spread. These represent worst case outcomes to compare other data against. Many other states, especially in the Midwest and the West, have not experienced high rates of increase in deaths relating to COVID-19. These states have flatter curves.

In general, the Midwest has fared quite well. The Minneapolis and St. Paul metro-region is no exception.[98] The top three most populous counties in Minnesota—Dakota, Hennepin, and Ramsey—reside within this region. All have managed to contain the spread. In Hennepin, the total number of deaths from the coronavirus has tended to double, at most, once every five days. Dakota and Ramsey have fared even better.

In Cook County, Illinois, home to the Windy City of Chicago, the

97 CDC. 2020. "Daily Updates of Totals by Week and State." *Centers for Disease Control and Prevention.*

98 Wikipedia. 2020. "Minneapolis–Saint Paul." *Wikipedia*, July 24.

rate of increase in cases and deaths has moderated, though officials are still uneasy about lifting restrictions.[99] Overall, the medical system in Illinois has successfully weathered the pandemic.[100] In my own state of North Dakota, the increase in fatalities from coronavirus has been even more modest. Health officials here have avidly traced transmission of the disease to ensure that it does not bring further disruption.[101] The relatively slow spread in these states is representative of outcomes in many other regions across the country.

Even in regions that have seen a modest increase in spread of coronavirus, the spread has been just that: modest. Medical systems across the Southwest are not overwhelmed and are largely expected to be able to handle any increase in patients from coronavirus.[102] Michigan and Louisiana have suffered the worst spread outside of the region of spread with New York as its epicenter.[103] There, estimated demand on ICUs exceeded capacity at the peak and have since fallen below capacity. In short, no region in the U.S. is currently experiencing a New York-like crisis.

---

99 Lewis, Sean, Elyse Russo, and Mike Ewing. 2020. "Chicago region falling short of reopening metrics, as Illinois' COVID-19 peak now expected in mid-June." *WGN9*, May 11.

100 IHME. 2020. "Illinois: Hospital Resource Use." *IHME COVID-19 Projections*.

101 Martin, Julie. 2020. "How North Dakota is tracking COVID-19 through contact tracing." *KFYRTV*, April 23.

102 IHME. 2020. "California: Hospital Resource Use," "Colorado: Hospital Resource Use," "New Mexico: Hospital Resource Use," "Arizona: Hospital Resource Use," "Nevada: Hospital Resource Use." *IHME COVID-19 Projections*.

103 IHME. 2020. "Michigan: Hospital Resource Use," "Louisiana: Hospital Resource Use." *IHME COVID-19 Projections*.

## NEW YORK AND NEARBY STATES

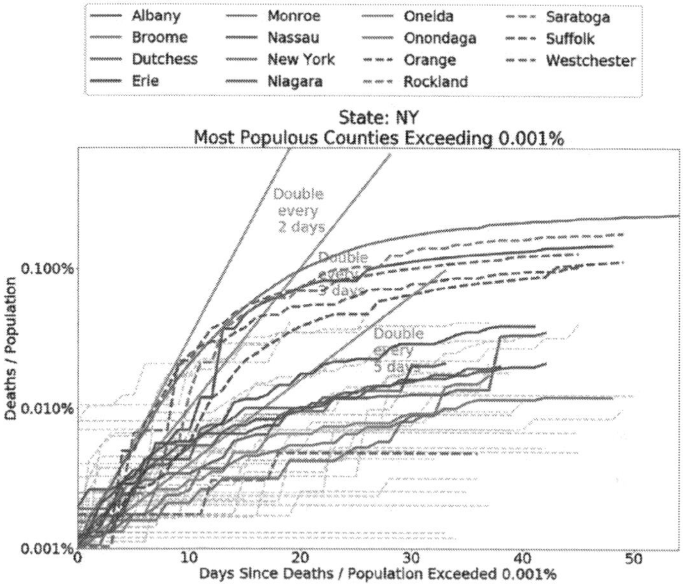


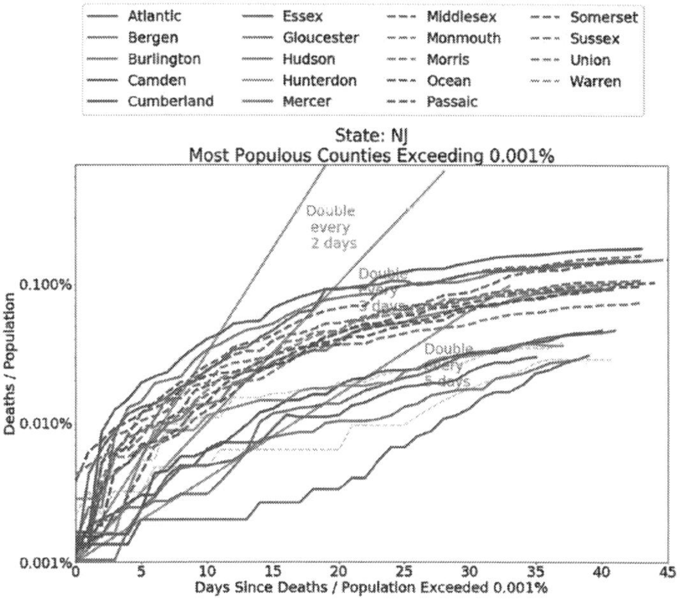

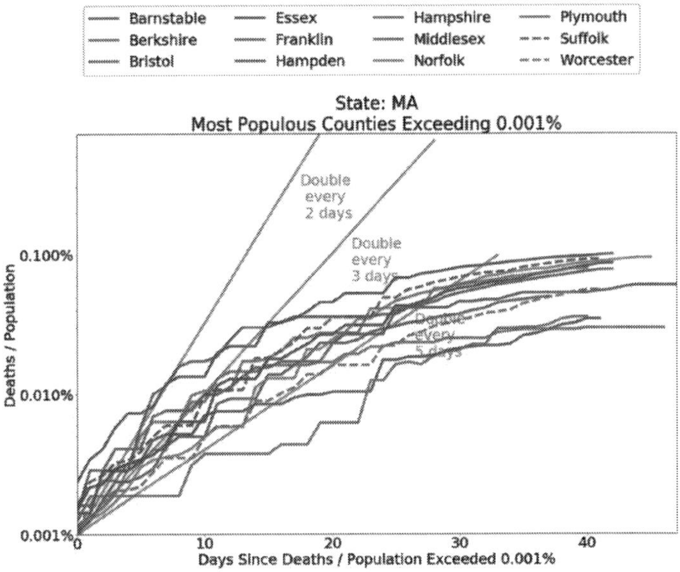
Barnstable
Berkshire
Bristol
Essex
Franklin
Hampden
Hampshire
Middlesex
Norfolk
Plymouth
Suffolk
Worcester
State: MA
Most Populous Counties Exceeding 0.001%
Double every 2 days
Double every 3 days
Double every 5 days
0.100%
0.010%
0.001%
Deaths / Population
0
10
20
30
40
Days Since Deaths / Population Exceeded 0.001%

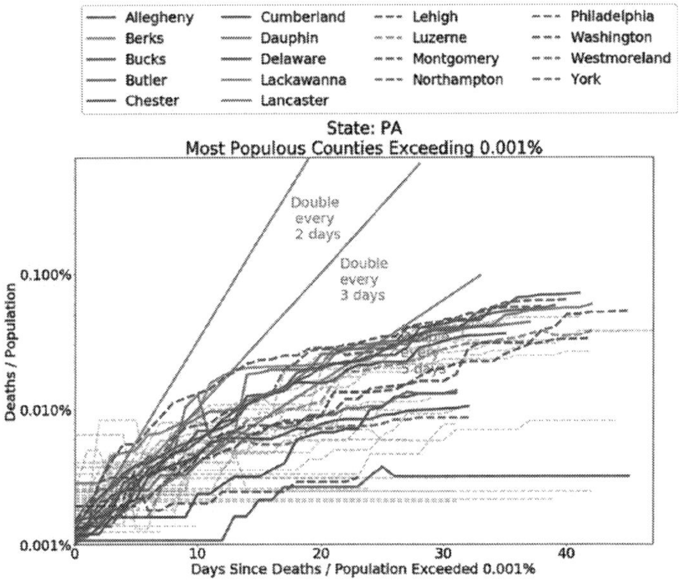
Allegheny
Berks
Bucks
Butler
Chester
Cumberland
Dauphin
Delaware
Lackawanna
Lancaster
Lehigh
Luzerne
Montgomery
Northampton
Philadelphia
Washington
Westmoreland
York
State: PA
Most Populous Counties Exceeding 0.001%
Double every 2 days
Double every 3 days
0.100%
0.010%
0.001%
Deaths / Population
0
10
20
30
40
Days Since Deaths / Population Exceeded 0.001%

## STATES IN OTHER REGIONS

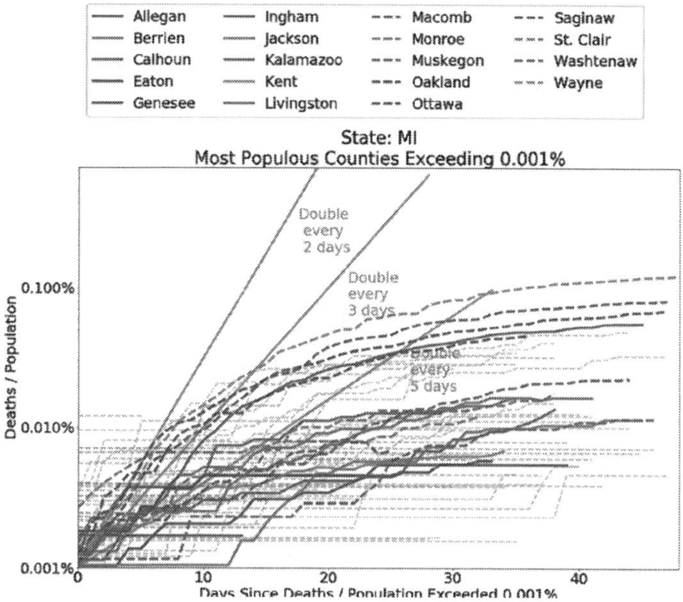


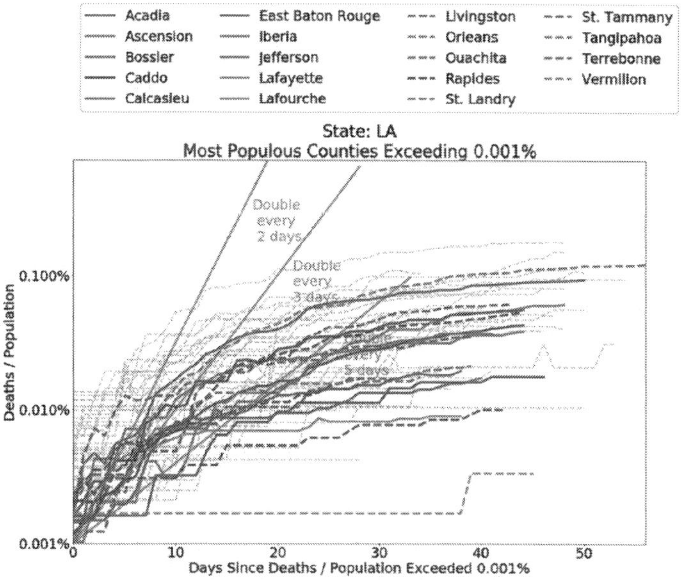

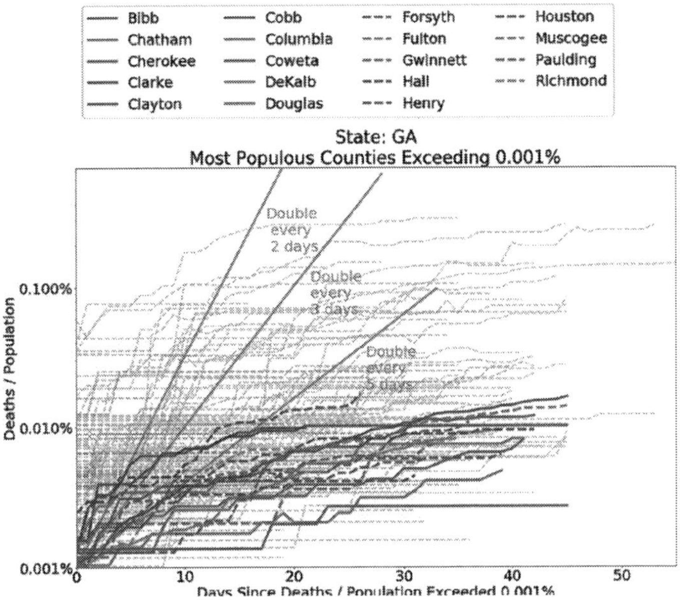
Bibb
Chatham
Cherokee
Clarke
Clayton
Cobb
Columbia
Coweta
DeKalb
Douglas
Forsyth
Fulton
Gwinnett
Hall
Henry
Houston
Muscogee
Paulding
Richmond
State: GA
Most Populous Counties Exceeding 0.001%
Double every 2 days
Double every 3 days
Double every 5 days
Deaths / Population
0.100%
0.010%
0.001%
0
10
20
30
40
50
Days Since Deaths / Population Exceeded 0.001%

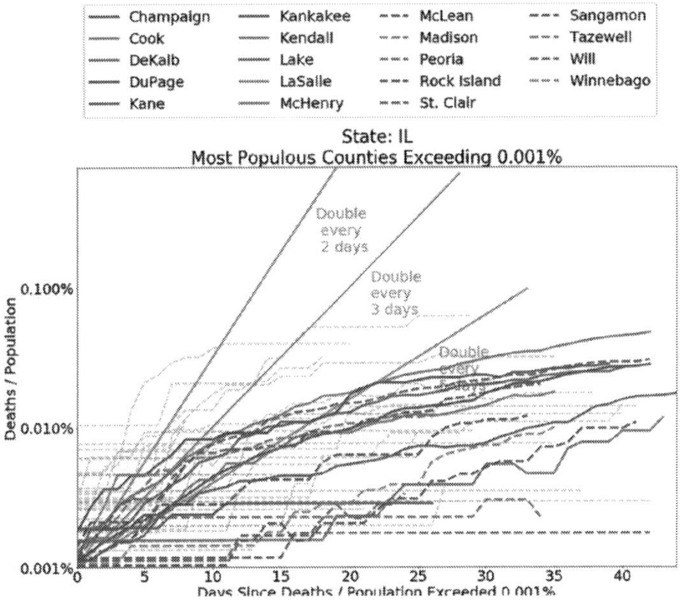
Champaign
Cook
DeKalb
DuPage
Kane
Kankakee
Kendall
Lake
LaSalle
McHenry
McLean
Madison
Peoria
Rock Island
St. Clair
Sangamon
Tazewell
Will
Winnebago
State: IL
Most Populous Counties Exceeding 0.001%
Double every 2 days
Double every 3 days
Deaths / Population
0.100%
0.010%
0.001%
0
5
10
15
20
25
30
35
40
Days Since Deaths / Population Exceeded 0.001%

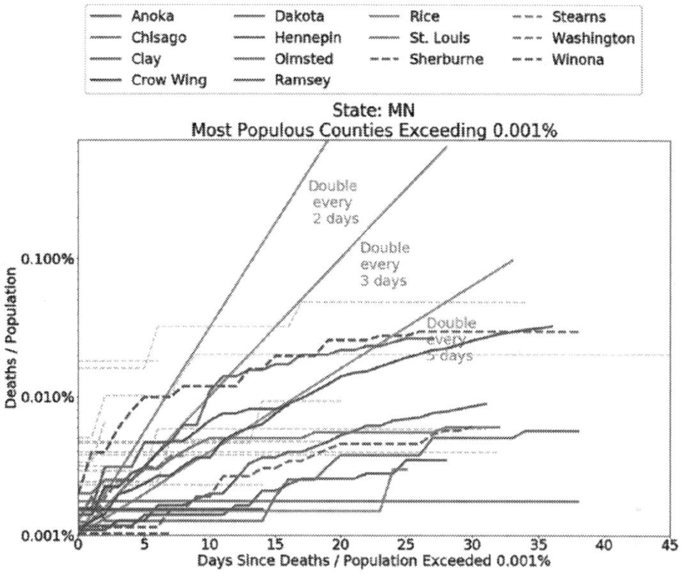
Anoka
Chisago
Clay
Crow Wing
Dakota
Hennepin
Olmsted
Ramsey
Rice
St. Louis
Sherburne
Stearns
Washington
Winona
State: MN
Most Populous Counties Exceeding 0.001%
Double every 2 days
Double every 3 days
Double every 5 days
Deaths / Population
0.100%
0.010%
0.001%
0
5
10
15
20
25
30
35
40
45
Days Since Deaths / Population Exceeded 0.001%

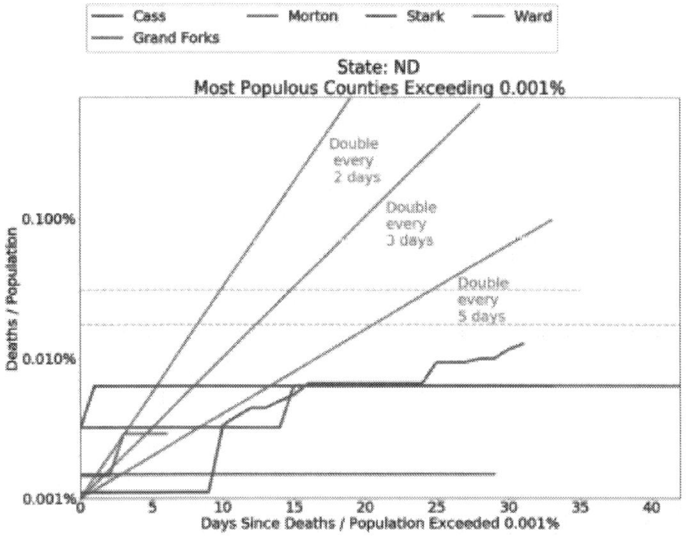
Cass
Grand Forks
Morton
Stark
Ward
State: ND
Most Populous Counties Exceeding 0.001%
Double every 2 days
Double every 3 days
Double every 5 days
Deaths / Population
0.100%
0.010%
0.001%
0
5
10
15
20
25
30
35
40
Days Since Deaths / Population Exceeded 0.001%

**Counties that rank in the top 20 most populous within each state *and* have measures of "Deaths / Population" ≥ 0.001% for COVID-19 related deaths are shown in solid. Counties outside of the top 20 are represented with dashed lines.[104] If a county does not appear on the map, "Deaths / Population" in that county is less than .001%.**

## AMERICA POST-LOCKDOWN

Given the continual stream of bad news that has bombarded the collective American consciousness over the last two months, it might be difficult to believe that the situation regarding the spread of COVID-19 is not dire, thanks in large part to the development of concern among the citizenry and a sense of corporate responsibility. Two weeks after many states have reopened, the new deaths and even the number of new cases across the country are still on the downtrend. While this is no time to throw caution to the wind, data seems to be a sign that our voluntary measures are succeeding.

Perhaps it is enough. Dr. Knut Wittowski, in his interview with AIER's president, Edward Stringham, advocates allowing for the coronavirus to spread among the healthy.[105] A faster spread will decrease the amount of time the vulnerable are at risk and, therefore, need to shelter.

The strategy worked in Sweden, which has fared about as well or better in terms of the percent of lives lost from COVID-19 than

---

104 Please visit www.aier.org/article/most-places-are-not-new-york-a-look-through-covid-19-data/ to view these graphs in color.

105 Stringham, Edward Peter. 2020. "Seminar with Edward Stringham, Knut Wittkowski, David Henderson, and Bill Luddy (Video)." *American Institute for Economic Research*, April 24; Stringham, Edward Peter. 2020. "Stand Up for Your Rights, says Bio-Statistician Knut M. Wittkowski." *American Institute for Economic Research*, April 6.

many of its neighbors that did lockdown.[106] The difference in the rate of spread of the virus in areas distant from New York suggest that the social distancing and hygienic measures have been effective. A diverse physical and social geography in the U.S. has also ensured that spread across most of the country has hardly been comparable to spread in New York.

If Americans let down their guard, we could see a second outbreak. While not outside of the realm of possibility, the slow rate of spread in states that did not issue stay-at-home-orders is an encouraging sign that COVID-19 is not ushering in an apocalypse.[107] Living in one of these states, I notice that even here people are especially careful. Aside from a limited number of establishments on Friday and Saturday evenings, the town is still quiet. Most people are staying home and, if they do go out, only ordering takeout. Most stores and restaurants that are open require that parties maintain social distancing protocol. In short, even in rural states, we have adapted.

It is a good thing that we have found voluntary means to approach the pandemic. Unemployment levels have pushed past 20%.[108] Every day the lockdown continues is another nail in the coffin for struggling American businesses and employees of those businesses. A collapse in

---

106 Caton, James L. 2020. "Beware a Second-Wave Attack on Liberty." *American Institute for Economic Research*, May 1; Book, Joakim. 2020. "What Sweden Has Done Right on Coronavirus." *American Institute for Economic Research*, March 31.

107 Cillizza, Chris. 2020. "7 governors still haven't issued stay-at-home orders. Here's why." *CNN*, April 13.

108 Hughes, Robert. 2020. "Massive Job Loss Sends Unemployment Rate to Highest Since the Great Depression." *American Institute for Economic Research*, May 8.

productivity has spelled the loss of livelihoods.[109] And with this loss, we will see more poverty. Tens of millions of Americans, and their families, are experiencing real suffering due the economic fallout that is accompanying the lockdown.[110] Layoffs have had a disproportionate effect on employment of workers with the lowest incomes.[111] To add to the difficulty, labor force participation has fallen by over 3 percent.[112] So much for the V-shaped recovery.

We cannot move on until much of the world has also moved on from this crisis. Disruption of supply chains around the world has shown us how closely bound together is our collective fate. Sweden may have avoided a shutdown, but it has not avoided an economic downturn.[113] Economic activity in one country is dependent upon the economic activity of its trading partners. Trade makes us rich because it allows each of us to provide value and offer it to others in the market. If half of the world is in lockdown, we are all poorer for it.

Perhaps this has been the cost of learning. Before the recent shutdown, contagious disease had passed from collective memory of America and much of the rest of the world. Yet the spread of a pathogen

---

109 Hughes, Robert. 2020. "May 2020 Business Conditions Monthly." *American Institute for Economic Research*, May 11.

110 Tucker, Jeffrey A. 2020. ""I've Lost Faith in Humanity": The Psychological Toll of the Lockdown." *American Institute for Economic Research*, April 28.

111 Beilfuss, Lisa. 2020. "Joblessness Is Soaring. Why Are Stocks Rising?" *Barron's*, May 8.

112 Stringham, Edward Peter. 2020. "A Tribute to the Wall Street Journal's Editorial Page." *American Institute for Economic Research*, May 11.

113 Ellyatt, Holly. 2020. "Sweden had no lockdown but its economy is expected to suffer just as badly as its European neighbors." *CNBC*, April 30.

like COVID-19 is not even a once-in-a-century event.[114] And at least as dangerous as COVID-19, a contagion of fear has swept the globe. We lacked an obvious contingency plan for protecting those vulnerable to disease, one that might guide us through troubled times.

Our problem was not that we did not shut down soon enough. As the experiences of Japan, South Korea, and Taiwan suggest, the shutdown of the economy is a sign of being ill-prepared.[115] Our problem was that we did not take the possibility of pandemic seriously. As we sensed the seriousness of the situation, we were not ready to take precaution appropriate to protect ourselves and those we love. Having learned, we need not fear.

---

114 Tucker, Jeffrey A. 2020. "Woodstock Occurred in the Middle of a Pandemic." *American Institute for Economic Research*, May 1.

115 Wikipedia. 2020. "COVID-19 pandemic in Japan." *Wikipedia*, July 24; Wikipedia. 2020. "COVID-19 pandemic in Taiwan." *Wikipedia*, July 24.

## FOCUS ON THE COVID-19 DEATH RATE

BY GREGORY VAN KIPNIS

May 24, 2020

In the saga of the virus and the lockdown, the wisdom of the crowds, that is the wisdom of each of us, was thwarted by bad data, perhaps intentionally bad. On the other hand, the ersatz wisdom of the collective bureaucracy in federal, state and local health agencies was based on crafted data. In the end data didn't matter, as the bureaucracies were more concerned with their natural territorial imperative, which is to rule and control.

The most frightening aspect of the novel coronavirus-19 (COVID-19) epidemic in the US is that it brought about exaggeratedly heightened fear of death. That fear, once magnified to proportions which become palpable to the individual, became the basis for dreadful economic and medical policies from governments and crushed the natural optimism of the public.

In early days, we were caught in a squeeze of conflicting information. Was COVID-19 a bioweapon gone rogue and destined to indiscriminately wipe out young and old? Or, was it another bad flu or perhaps an extremely bad flu? After all, initial information showed the victims were concentrated in a nursing home in Kirkland, Washington.

No cases were reported amongst the homeless on West Coast streets. No deaths among children were reported. And in the closed world of cruise liners and later a military ship, there were lots of early cases and some deaths. As time passed, there was little more bad news. We should have been suspicious of the data.

We were mainly focused on the case fatality rate which were

frighteningly high.[116] We worried about the infection fatality rate, but there was too little data and testing available to have any idea how many people were or ultimately would be infected.[117]

But those concepts—CFR and IFR—are not the most important strategic measures of the severity of the disease. It is the death rate, properly defined and understood, that should matter for long-term policy makers, our erstwhile more level-headed thinkers, in determining policy.

In the past few weeks, we have obtained more useful data in the US. There were secrets lurking in the data, waiting to be uncovered, that could help ascertain what was really happening. The purpose of this report is to do just that—to ascertain what the data are telling us. It also gives us the basis for judging the appropriateness of past and present policies.

So, let's begin with a simple question: what is the relevant death rate due to COVID-19? There are many definitions in the epidemiological world such as the CFR and IFR mentioned above. My focus is on the overall death rate—actual and projected. Until we have more widespread testing for COVID-19, we cannot know with any accuracy how many people were infected by the virus. We cannot know what proportion of the population has some sort of natural or acquired immunity.

We do not even have accurate data on how many people have died from COVID-19 alone versus COVID-19 plus some other complications that were already present such as diabetes, morbid obesity and

---

116 CFR: deaths as a percent of diagnosed cases.

117 IFR: deaths as a percent of diagnosed and undiagnosed cases.

prior respiratory complications, any one of which might equally have been the proximate cause of death. There is ample evidence, especially in the Northeast region that there has been "over classification" (a euphemism for data bias). We do not have the demographic details for those infected and those who died. But we do have death data, and it is more accurate than the number of cases and the number of infections.

To understand how our minds have been misdirected in understanding the real risks associated with COVID-19, let's begin with a brain teaser. It will awaken our numerate minds in preparation for understanding the data deception and misunderstandings that prevail.

## WHEN IS 1.7% GREATER THAN 98.3%?

In the bizarro world of COVID-19 reporting that is the case—1.7% is greater than 98.3%. Specifically, deaths among a narrow 1.7% group of the population are greater than deaths from the other 98.3%. Numerically a death may be a death, but from a policy point of view, to be blunt about it, not all deaths are the same. **Fact #1:** 1.7% of the population in the US resides in long-term medical care facilities (LTMCFs) and total 5.7 million. **Fact #2:** The residents of LTMCFs accounted for 38,800 or 53% of all COVID-19 deaths (based on recent data). The rest of the country, the 98.3%, have experienced approximately 34,600 deaths, or 47% of the nation's total COVID-19 deaths.

## THE DEATH RATE AT LTMCFS IS STUNNING

That means the death rate, deaths expressed as a percent of those living in medical care institutions, is 0.682%, more than 50 times the death rate of the rest of the population at 0.012%. The death rate for the overall populations is 0.022%.

That should leave you speechless.

We have a COVID-19 problem, but we have an even greater and more serious LTMCF problem that is clouding our understanding of the contagion and therefore what our best public health policies should be. Shutting down the economy, the world wherein the 98.3% live and prosper was too draconian. The feared overloading of the hospital system with emergency patients, which was short-lived, was disproportionately coming from the residents of LTMCFs, not the general public.

The data have been there all along, but they were not properly collected, catalogued and analyzed.

Much of the data in this report came from a landmark study by Gregg Girvan and Avik Roy of the Foundation for Research of Equal Opportunity.[118] Their work was based on data collected through May 10th 2020 for most states. Since their publication, revisions have been incorporated as states have corrected or updated their data since the original report. The calculations given above are imputations from the updated data.

At this point, we do not know what the ultimate count of deaths and the death rate will be, but what wc havc in hand arc statistics that are very indicative and telling of the gross misunderstanding that the public and federal, state and local decision-makers have been working with on which to base their decisions.

Long-term medical care providers to the aged and medically infirm (per the Girvan-Roy study) consist of: nursing homes and skilled nursing facilities; assisted living facilities (i.e., residential care

---

118 Girvan, Gregg. 2020. "Nursing Homes & Assisted Living Facilities Account for 45% of COVID-19 Deaths." *FREOPP*, May 7.

communities or personal care homes); adult day service centers; home health agencies; and hospices.

The first two medical care providers for seniors are referred to as long-term medical care facilities (LTMCF) and are the source of the data. Data for the other three elder care facilities are not collected or were not available for the Girvan-Roy study. In fact, it has been acknowledged that there continues to be underreporting of deaths related to LTMCFs. Some providers are just not reporting. In other cases, the residents die in hospitals and they are not categorized as LTMCF deaths. Nonetheless, the data are sufficient to draw some useful if not stark observations.

## WHAT ABOUT THE FLU AND PNEUMONIA DEATH RATES IN EARLIER YEARS?

To even better understand these death rate figures, it is useful to put them into the context of what we know about death rates from the flu before the arrival of COVID-19. Is the COVID-19 death rate worse, better or about the same as prior flu seasons? We should expect the rates to be worse because there is no vaccine whereas most people get a vaccine shot for routine flus that are expected each year.

In 2017 the Centers for Disease Control (CDC) reported that annual deaths from all causes were 2.8 million or 0.866% of the population. The leading causes of death, in order of magnitude, were heart disease, cancer, accidents, respiratory disease, stroke, Alzheimer's disease, diabetes, flu & pneumonia and suicide.

Just looking at the Flu & Pneumonia (FP) cause, in 2017 it accounted for 55,672 deaths or 0.017% for the population as a whole.[119] Death

---

119 CDC. 2019. "Deaths: Leading Causes for 2017." *National Vital Statistics Reports*, June 24, 68(6).

from FP, as you would expect, fell hardest on people over 75 totaling 38,078 deaths. That translates into a FP death rate of 0.180% for those over-75 group, which is a little more than 10 times the death rate for the overall population. For the rest of the population under 75 the death rate was only 0.006%, or or 1/30th of those over 75 (0.006% vs 0.180%).

DEATH RATE FOR COVID-19 AND THE FLU FOR SELECTED DEMOGRAPHICS

| | 2020 COVID-19 | 2017 Flu & Pneumonia |
|---|---|---|
| Overall Death Rate | 0.022% | 0.017% |
| Over 75 DR | 0.161% | 0.180% |
| LTMCFs DR | 0.682% | |
| Non-LTMCFs DR | 0.011% | |
| Under 75 DR | 0.010% | 0.006% |

*Data from CDC and FreeOpp.*

What this means at this point is that in the aggregate the overall COVID-19 death rate is slightly worse than the flu death rate in a prior year (0.022% vs 0.017%). However, for seniors in LTMCFs, the COVID-19 death rate is 100 times greater than the flu and pneumonia DR was for those under 75 in 2017 (0.682% vs 0.006%) and nearly 4 times greater than those over 75.

In summary the COVID-19 death rate is far more skewed to those older than 75 and those residents in medical care facilities for the aged.

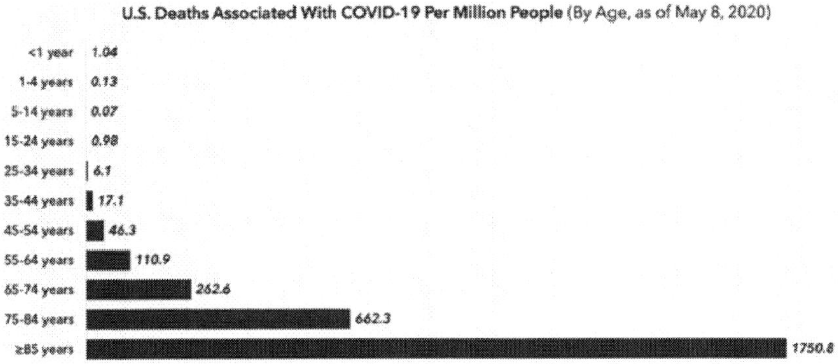


The risk of death from COVID-19 is far higher in the elderly than in younger Americans. According to data from the Centers for Disease Control and Prevention, there have been 23 deaths associated with COVID-19 per million people among those aged 25 to 54, whereas there have been 566 deaths per million among those over 65: a 25-fold difference. Note that not all COVID-19 deaths reported elsewhere are counted by CDC, and that not all CDC-counted deaths were caused by COVID-19; some of these individuals died from other causes, but tested positive for SARS-CoV-2 antibodies. If we assume that there will be 120,000 total deaths from COVID-19 in the U.S., the odds of an individual under 25 dying from COVID-19 are around 1.6 per million, or 1 in 633,000. (Graphics: A. Ray / FREOPP)

Looking ahead we obtained the most recent forecast from the Institute for Health Metrics and Evaluation (IHME) at the University of Washington. They are considered by many medical professionals as the most thorough modelers. On May 18, 2020 the IHME released the results of the third run of its new model. They predict that by August 4, 2020 a total of 143,357 Americans will die of COVID-19. That forecast nearly doubles the number of COVID-19 deaths. It is worth noting that each run of the model has produced lower forecasts for future deaths. There are detractors of their modeling procedures, but it is the best we have at the moment.

One interesting medical research report suggests that a significant portion of the population has natural immunity to COVID-19. Researchers found:[120]

120 Grifoni, Alba, Daniela Weiskopf, Sydney I. Ramirez, Jose Mateus, Jennifer M. Dan et al. 2020. "Targets of T Cell Responses to SARS-CoV-2 Coronavirus in Humans with COVID-19 Disease and Unexposed Individuals." *Cell*, 181(7): 1489-1501.

> T cell responses were detected in 40-60% of unexposed individuals. This may be reflective of some degree of cross-reactive, preexisting immunity to SARSCoV-2 in some, but not all, individuals... suggesting cross-reactive T cell recognition between circulating 'common cold' coronaviruses and SARS-CoV-2.

This might be why there are so many reports of asymptomatic cases of COVID-19. That also may mean the IHME forecast will be revised down even more.

However, COVID-19 has brutal consequences for people over 75. That detail cannot be minimized. But what policies would that suggest?

## DID WE ADOPT THE RIGHT POLICIES?

What do these data suggest about the medical and economic policies that have been adopted by the federal, states and local governments?

The carnage of COVID-19 is concentrated in elder care facilities not in the population at large. The policies and procedures, including lockdowns and state-of-the-art personal protection practices for those facilities, should have been more thoroughly thought out based on useful data.

Keep in mind, about 70% of the elder care facilities are for-profit. Yet they are not free-market enterprises; enterprises free to do what they think is best. These for-profit facilities are licensed and regulated by the several Departments of Health of the states. They do what the state tells them to do.

The governors and mayors, and their medical and science advisers, made the decision to pack them in, force them to house and retain infected and returning infected patients. They chose to divert PPE supplies to hospitals, not the elder care facilities. This characterization is based on reports in the press. One certainly hopes there were some communities that did a better job. There is reason to believe that is the case because some assisted living facilities have reported no deaths.

As COVID-19 deaths mounted, not a word was officially spoken about where they were occurring. Fear was stoked that it was a population-wide epidemic. We should ALL lock down.

What a costly mistake, a mistake that continues to this day. Governors and mayors with fresh data insights into the truth still want to be central planners and determine which businesses can re-open and to what degree, who should still shelter or socially distance. They send out teams to draw circles in the grass defining where groups can camp out and place police monitors in all the parks to warn people to stay within the circles. At this point they are just imaginary prisons, but they are prisons.

Madness, sheer madness.

Though that is an easy and superficial observation to make, what is really unsaid, and not easy to admit, is that large numbers of politicians and bureaucrats have revealed their true nature. Speeches decorated with declarations of "better safe than sorry" and "planning is better than no planning" reveal they are authoritarians by nature; central planners of the worst kind.

In conclusion, the relevant death rate for policy purposes has been obscured. The consequence has been inappropriate policies. They have resulted in a bizarro world of highly restricted commercial functioning and immense economic destruction, alongside no evidence that lives were saved and growing evidence of second-tier loss of life resulting from lockdown.

## THE REAL PANDEMIC WAS A NURSING HOME PROBLEM

BY PETER C. EARLE

June 30, 2020

Over the last week, many governors have reinstituted coronavirus policy implementations which had been in various phases of cessation. Why? This is because of an alleged "spike" in new COVID-19 infections.[121] Other states have abbreviated their phased lifting of lockdowns. This is despite the fact that current US deaths from COVID-19 are now 90% off their peak.

Washington State is considering criminalizing the refusal to wear a mask.[122] New York State governor Andrew Cuomo has imposed new out-of-state visitor bans with the comment that: "in addition to law enforcement, [he] … expect[s] individuals such as hotel clerks … to question travelers from select states."[123] Democratic Presidential candidate Joe Biden's comments that if he were to win the presidency, a federal mask mandate may follow.[124] The Speaker of the House quickly voiced her support for that measure.[125]

---

121 Miller, Stephen. 2020. "What Spike? Hospitalization Data Show No Indication of a Second Wave." *American Institute for Economic Research*, June 16.

122 Cohen, Li. 2020. "Washington state to require face masks after county runs out of hospital beds." *CBS News*, June 24.

123 Spiering, Charlie. 2020. "Gov. Andrew Cuomo: Police May Stop Cars with Out-of-State Plates to Enforce Quarantine." *Breitbart*, June 24.

124 Stracqualursi, Veronica, and Sarah Mucha. 2020. "Biden says he would make wearing face masks mandatory for Americans amid coronavirus pandemic." *CNN Politics*, June 26.

125 Wise, Alana. 2020. "Nancy Pelosi Calls Trump 'Cowardly' For Not Wearing Mask, Supports Federal Mandate." *NPR*, June 26.

These and other developments suggest that rather than approaching the end of the government-created crisis, we may be at the threshold of a new beginning. That the recent rise in infections is mostly an artifact of massively expanded testing capabilities seems to occur to no one in the government or media. Equally unnoticed is that the apparently much wider spread of COVID-19 infections, many of which show middling symptoms or are treated as annoyances, should result in a decrease of concern: it appears that many times the number of people estimated early on as infected by the novel coronavirus have been to little or no consequence.[126]

And further still, that some of the spike is accountable to the civil unrest in the wake of the murder of George Floyd. The prevalence of new COVID-19 infections among mostly Gen-Zs and Millennials (beside their prevalence in jobs that require COVID testing, such as in the fast food and service industries) undoubtedly had much to do with the disingenuity of political officials who ordered them to stay home, out of work and away from social occasions, yet responded with deafening silence as protests, demonstrations, and rioting broke out.

Note the recent data trend in California:[127]

| California | 7-Jun | 18-Jun | 28-Jun | | New cases, 6/18 to 6/28 | % of new cases with age knov |
|---|---|---|---|---|---|---|
| <5 | 1826 | 2703 | 3854 | | 1151 | 2.25% |
| Age 5-17 | 6422 | 9360 | 13303 | | 3943 | 7.71% |
| 18-34 | 36930 | 48742 | 68070 | | 19328 | 37.79% |
| 35-49 | 32985 | 41536 | 54763 | | 13227 | 25.86% |
| 50-59 | 21394 | 26231 | 32859 | | 6628 | 12.96% |
| 60-64 | 8631 | 10254 | 12575 | | 2321 | 4.54% |
| 65-69 | 6265 | 7377 | 8895 | | 1518 | 2.97% |
| 70-74 | 4698 | 5417 | 6495 | | 1078 | 2.11% |
| 75-79 | 3621 | 4148 | 4855 | | 707 | 1.38% |
| 80+ | 8355 | 9443 | 10684 | | 1241 | 2.43% |

126 Etherington, Darrell. 2020. “Color’s COVID-19 testing shows most who test positive had either mild or no symptoms.” *TechCrunch*, June 15.

127 CDPH. 2020. “Cases and Deaths Associated with COVID-19 by Age Group in California.” *California Department of Public Health*, July 22.

Or in Minnesota:[128]

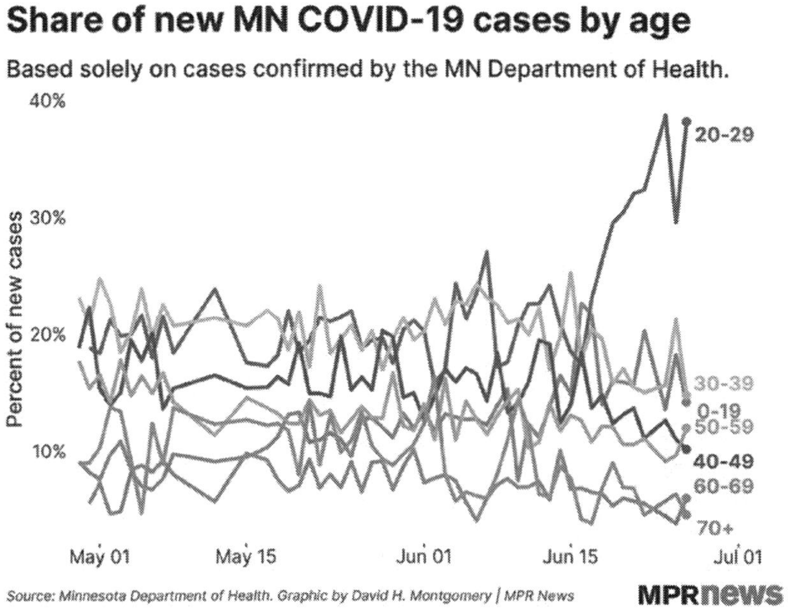


As other statistics regarding the toll of the novel coronavirus outbreak firm up, certain patterns are beginning to come into focus. With increasing certainty we can say that locked down states have seen four times the death toll of non-locked down states.[129] The effectiveness of masking is, as well, being revealed as suspect, as is social distancing in the absence of testing and contact tracing.[130]

---

128 MPR News Staff. 2020. "June 28 update on COVID-19 in MN: Outbreak appears to be plateauing in recent days." *MPR News*, June 28.

129 Stringham, Edward Peter. 2020. "Again, What Were the Benefits of Locking Down?" *American Institute for Economic Research*, June 25.

130 The efficacy of contact tracing is additionally questionable. See article herein entitled "Doubts About Contact Tracing."

A more important revelation of the ongoing deluge of data has been either missed (or ignored) by the press. At AIER, we noted the stunning death rates in long-term care facilities back in the third week of May.[131]

Just a few days ago, the *New York Times* reported that 54,000 deaths due to COVID-19—43% of all deaths in the United States—occurred in nursing home residents and workers:[132]

> In 24 states, the number of residents and workers who have died accounts for either half or more than half of all deaths from the virus. Infected people linked to nursing homes also die at a higher rate than the general population. The median case fatality rate—the number or deaths divided by the number of cases—at facilities with reliable data is 17 percent, significantly higher than the 5 percent fatality rate nationwide.

New York State was only one of several states, though, which enacted orders increasing the virus death tolls.[133]

> States that issued orders similar to Cuomo's recorded comparably grim outcomes. Michigan lost 5% of roughly 38,000 nursing home residents to COVID-19 since the outbreak began. New Jersey lost 12% of its more than 43,000 residents. In

131 See article herein entitled "Focus on the COVID-19 Death Rate."

132 NYT. 2020. "More Than 40% of U.S. Coronavirus Deaths Are Linked to Nursing Homes." *The New York Times*, July 15.

133 Sapien, Joaquin, and Joe Sexton. 2020. "'Fire Through Dry Grass': Andrew Cuomo Saw COVID-19's Threat to Nursing Homes. Then He Risked Adding to It." *ProPublica*, June 16.

> Florida, where such transfers were barred, just 1.6% of 73,000 nursing home residents died of the virus. California, after initially moving toward a policy like New York's, quickly revised it. So far, it has lost 2% of its 103,000 nursing home residents.

And keep in mind that this 43% average is massively dragged down because five states had zero deaths in nursing homes while other states had as many of 80% of their deaths in nursing homes.

**Cases and deaths in long-term care facilities, by state**

| | FACILITIES | CASES | DEATHS | SHARE OF COVID-19 DEATHS ▼ |
|---|---|---|---|---|
| United States | 12,000 | 282,000 | 54,000 | **43%** |
| New Hampshire | 26 | 1,967 | 293 | **80%** |
| Rhode Island | 64 | 2,745 | 715 | **77%** |
| Minnesota | 853 | 5,777 | 1,107 | **77%** |
| Connecticut | 289 | 9,888 | 3,124 | **73%** |
| Pennsylvania | 678 | 20,689 | 4,518 | **68%** |
| North Dakota | 65 | 569 | 56 | **64%** |
| Massachusetts | 565 | 23,321 | 5,115 | **64%** |
| Idaho | 30 | 323 | 56 | **62%** |
| Maryland | 289 | 12,641 | 1,924 | **61%** |
| Virginia | 236 | 6,714 | 1,039 | **61%** |
| Kentucky | 172 | 2,626 | 350 | **61%** |
| Washington | 389 | 4,376 | 779 | **60%** |
| Vermont | 6 | 172 | 32 | **57%** |
| Ohio | 530 | 9,928 | 1,580 | **57%** |

Source: *New York Times*

This development is magnified in its awfulness upon close inspection of the document which informed the lockdown policies. The second-to-last paragraph in the original 2006 *Nature* article—the blueprint for the lockdowns, entitled "Strategies for Mitigating an Influenza Pandemic" reads,

> Lack of data prevent us from reliably modeling transmission in the important context of residential institutions (for example, care homes, prisons) and health care settings; detailed planning for use of antivirals, vaccines, and infection control measures in such settings are needed, however. We do not present projections of the likely impact of personal protective measures (for example, face masks) on transmission, again due to a lack of data on effectiveness.

The apparent omission of considerations regarding individuals in long-term care facilities by epidemiologists and policymakers, and the consequently disproportionate number of total fatalities among that same population, provides context for a series of hasty, surreptitious actions by politicians to duck accountability (and harvest more power).[134]

It thus becomes increasingly clear that despite driving the U.S. economy into an artificial depression, destroying tens of thousands

---

134 Phillips, Morgan. 2020. "Cuomo says 'nobody' should be prosecuted over coronavirus deaths amid criticism over nursing home policy." *Fox News*, May 18; 2020. "In March, Cuomo Quietly Slipped In Liability Protections To Shield Hard-Hit Nursing Homes From Lawsuits." *Kaiser Health News*, May 14; Schultz, Marisa. 2020. "Cuomo attempts to deflect blame of deadly nursing home coronavirus debacle on to Trump." *Fox News*, May 23; Sirota, David. 2020. "Cuomo gave immunity to nursing home executives after big campaign donations." *The Guardian*, May 26.

of businesses and the lives of millions of citizens, and elevating rates of domestic violence, divorce, substance abuse, and suicide, US government policies failed to protect the most vulnerable segment of the population: individuals in nursing homes and other long-term care facilities.[135] And furthermore, that despite 14 years between the publication of the "Strategies" paper and its real-world implementation, apparently no research was conducted that would have extended its conclusions to those particularly at-risk populations.

This, of course, is a vastly more fundamental issue than the inability of even the most complex computational methods to incorporate and account for social science phenomena. The susceptibility of the elderly and institutionalized, and in particular those with pre-existing conditions, was a ubiquitous consideration of virtually all medical protocols. Yet somehow between the 1970s and today, human knowledge regarding disease prevention and control—a product of informal institutions and cultural mores—was lost or forgotten; and into the vacuum swept the rigidities of top-down edicts informed by

---

135 Tucker, Hank. 2020. "Coronavirus Bankruptcy Tracker: These Major Companies Are Failing Amid The Shutdown." *Forbes*, May 3; Durden, Tyler. 2020. "41% Of Business Closures On Yelp Have Permanently Closed As V-Shaped Recovery Implodes." *ZeroHedge*, June 28; McMickle, John. 2020. "The calm before the storm of bankruptcies." *American Banker*, June 15; Ziv, Shaher. 2020. "Don't Be Fooled By Official Unemployment Rate Of 14.7%; The Real Figure Is Even Scarier." *Forbes*, May 10; Kaplan, Adiel, and Wilson Wong. 2020. "It's hard to flee from your domestic abuser during a coronavirus lockdown." *NBC News*, May 17; Kingkade, Tyler. 2020. "Police see rise in domestic violence calls amid coronavirus lockdown." *NBC News*, April 5; Fies, Andy. 2020. "Surge in divorces anticipated in wake of COVID-19 quarantine." *ABC News*, April 17; Polakovic, Gary. 2020. "Pandemic drives alcohol sales—and raises concerns about substance abuse." *USC News*, April 14; Thakyr, Vikram, and Anu Jain. 2020. "COVID 2019-suicides: A global psychological pandemic." *Brain, Behavior and Immunity*, S0889-1591(20): 30643-7.

scientism: technocrats wielding agent-based models.

Americans expect government agencies to lie and their prognoses and diagnoses to fail.[136] Policy failures are vastly more common than successes, and successes—where they may be found—are always and everywhere a veritable font of unintended consequences.

Far from producing better responses, models and simulations used as detailed outlines (rather than for high-level, mostly abstract insights) amplify, rather than attenuate, the failures of central planning. The model-driven response to the coronavirus pandemic, which now includes directly sacrificing the most vulnerable segment of the population to the virus, is only the latest. And it joins a growing heap of episodes which include the Fed's response to the late 1920s financial boom and more recently the destruction of Iraq over WMDs that scarcely existed and the botched emergency response to Hurricane Katrina.

Why do we continue to listen?

---

136 Pew Research. 2019. "Public Trust in Government: 1958-2019." *Pew Research Centre*, April 11; Montanaro, Domenico. 2020. "Poll: Americans Don't Trust What They're Hearing From Trump On Coronavirus." *NPR*, March 17.

## WHY WE SHOULD NOT BE CONCERNED ABOUT INCREASING COVID-19 CASES IN TEXAS

BY EDWARD P. STRINGHAM

July 2, 2020

Should we be concerned about the total number of COVID-19 *deaths* or COVID-19 *cases* that do not result in death? On June 29, 2020, former *New York Times* reporter Alex Berenson, and an important alternative voice on COVID-19, received a note from a managing partner of the medical care facilities CompleteCare in Texas.[137] The author tells of what's happening on the ground, and it differs dramatically from the headlines driving Texas officials to once again close up the economy in a panic over a rise in cases.

Recall that the original idea of "flattening the curve" was not to make the virus go away but to slow the spread of infections to prevent hospitals from getting overwhelmed in the short run.[138] The stay-at-home order for two weeks was meant to buy time for hospitals to get enough equipment and deal with patients over time rather than all at once. The good news is the hospitals were never overrun.

It also turns out that COVID-19 deaths were a fraction of the most alarmist predictions that drove public policy, and over time COVID-19 deaths continue to decrease.

But now we hear about rising cases—not deaths—and that is introducing more calls for lockdowns and travel bans.

What the letter reports will not shock anyone who has followed

---

137 Berenson, Alex (@AlexBerensen). 2020. "Wondering what's really happening in Texas? Here's the email[...]" *Twitter*, June 29, 2020.

138 This was never an issue in Texas.

cases during the reopening period. The cases are mostly young people who are in very little danger from the virus. What should be considered good news—that the case fatality rate is falling each day—is being misinterpreted by the press.

As for this gentleman's willingness to speak out, it is a heroic act in these strange times. He worries of becoming a target—which is a legitimate concern. Even so, the truth needs to come out. AIER gives the letter, originally posted on Berenson's twitter feed, a full airing.

> Good morning,
>
> I am the Managing Partner and General Counsel of a Texas based company that owns and operates 13 free-standing emergency clinics in the State of Texas. I follow your reporting and wanted to share with you some information on Texas. I want people to hear this story as opposed to the mainstream reporting. However, I am sensitive about putting a target on myself or my company for conveying this information. I am not sure how you've handled this type of situation but I suspect you've had other people send you information who are concerned about becoming a target.
>
> In June, we tested over 2,231 patients (data through last Thursday). **Positive rate is now close to 20% (was 4-6% in May). Vast majority of the cases are mild to very mild symptoms. Average age of the people getting tested in mid-30s.**
>
> Very different patient (in terms of age) than we've seen before June. Most of these patients would not have met criteria that we previously had (and all the health facilities had) for Covid testing. Now with more testing kits we are able to test a broader group of patients.

Clinically, we've had very few hospital transfers because of Covid. **Vast majority of the patients are better within 2-3 days of the visit and most would be described as having a cold (a mild one at that) or the symptoms related to allergies.** We've often provided a steroid shot and some antibiotics. **By the time we have follow-up calls, most of the patients are no longer experiencing any symptoms.** They often say the shot really made a difference.

In terms of what is driving them to the ER—**Roughly 1/2 have been told by their employers to get a test. They have a sneeze or a cough and their employer tells them to go get tested.** The other 1/2 just want to know. They have mild symptoms (and some don't have any symptoms but game the system and check a box that they have a symptom so they can get a test—they cannot get a test unless they present with symptoms. If they have no symptoms we send them away—which does happen.)

**The average length of stay of Covid patients is 3-5 days.** Much lower than the patients being seen in April and early May. Their symptoms are also milder. **Most of the patients are not ending up in the ICU. The hospital ICUs are filled with really sick people with non-Covid issues. They [didn't] come in earlier because they were scared and now they are super sick.** From multiple sources at different hospitals—they have plenty of capacity and no shortage of acute care beds.

No real data on breakdown of patients who have Covid but are not in the hospital because of Covid. Recognition that because all patients are tested for Covid you have some percentage of patients listed as Covid patients who are non Covid

> symptomatic and that the hospitalization rate is somewhat driven by hospitals taking their normal patients with other medical issues.
>
> Finally, heard several stories of how **discharge planners are being pressured to put Covid as primary diagnosis—as that pays significantly better.** Hospitals want to avoid the discussion but if they don't they risk another shutdown. This may be an explanation for why there is a gap in hospital executives saying they have plenty of capacity and the increasing number of Covid hospitalizations. **You open up your hospitals for normal medical care and you test everyone (sic) of those patients—the result is higher percentage of patients who have Covid—now.**
>
> Overall, based on what we are seeing at our facilities, the above information is really a positive story. **You have more people testing positive with really minimal symptoms. This means that the fatality rate is less than commonly reported.**

Thus do we have first-hand confirmation of what we've suspected. So many of the new cases are among the young and so many of those infected have no symptoms or mild symptoms.

Previously we had less capacity to do testing and so many people with COVID-19 went undiagnosed. Now that we are doing more testing, more people who would have been undiagnosed are being diagnosed. Thus the upward trend in diagnosed cases. But the good news is that the deaths continue to decrease even as we find more previously undiagnosed cases.

This chart shows weekly death counts by age over the past few months. These decreases should be cause for cheer rather than cause for more lockdown.

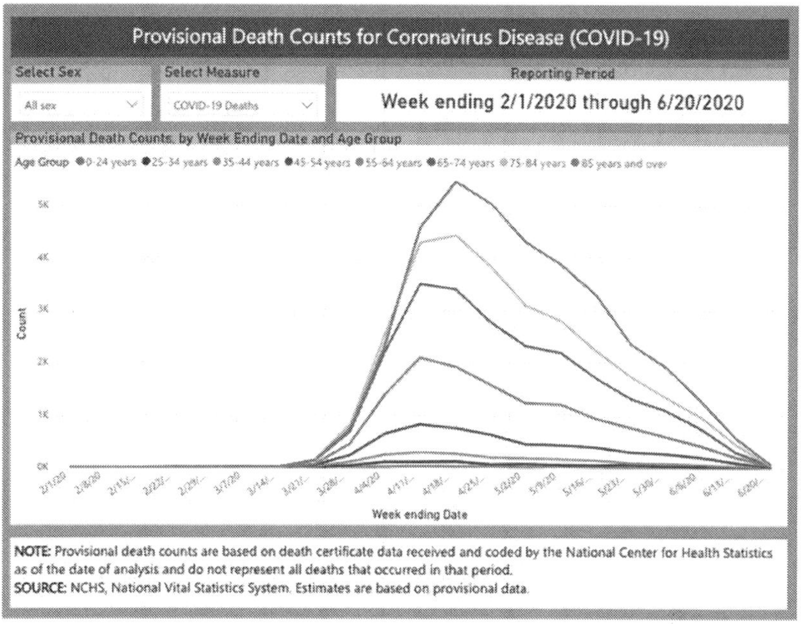


CDC. 2020. "Provisional Death Counts for Coronavirus Disease (COVID-19)." *CDC*, July 22.

It turns out that COVID-19 has a much lower fatality rate, especially among young people, when we include all of the previously undiagnosed cases.

The Centers for Disease Control Director Robert R. Redfield now estimates that about 20 million Americans have had and have recovered from COVID-19. That means this deadly disease does not have a fatality rate of 6 percent but of 0.6 percent. And among young people the fatality rate is magnitudes lower than that.

The fact that increased testing means we are discovering more young and healthy people with COVID-19 should not be surprising or alarming in the slightest.

The hospitals are under financial pressure from having to mostly stop doing business for months, so they are classifying as many people as possible as a COVID case in order to take advantage of federal government subsidies. Overall, this is good news. Somehow, this is being spun as some kind of disaster that once again requires shutting down.

## DON'T LET HOSPITALIZATION TRENDS BLIND YOU TO THE NUMBERS THEMSELVES

BY STEPHEN C. MILLER

July 3, 2020

Since I wrote about hospitalizations two weeks ago, the trend in current hospitalizations has reversed, with more COVID hospitalizations now than there were a month ago, although still well below the peak in mid-April.[139]

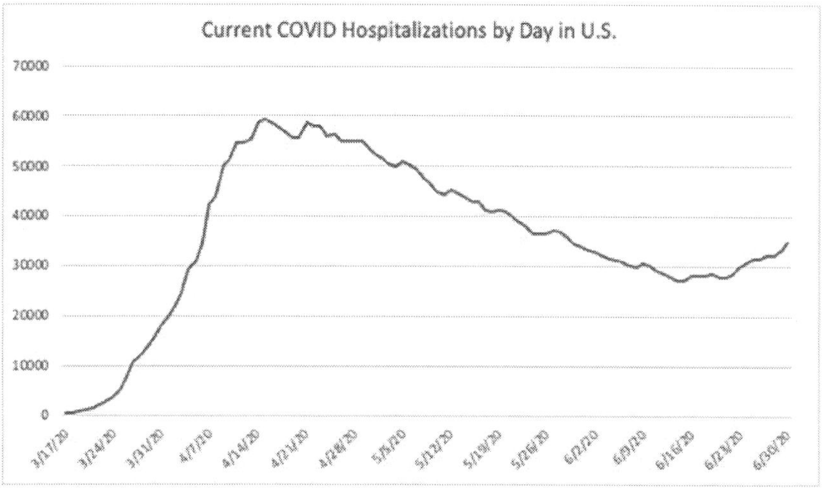


The trend in *new* hospitalizations nationally, is still flat, as the next chart shows. Not only is the recent trend flat, but the current weekly average of new hospitalizations is lower than it was one, two, and even three months ago.[140]

---

139 Miller, Stephen C. 2020. "What Spike? Hospitalization Data Show No Indication of a Second Wave." *American Institute for Economic Research*, June 16.

140 The data used in this article were downloaded from *The Atlantic*'s COVID Tracking Project on July 1st 2020.

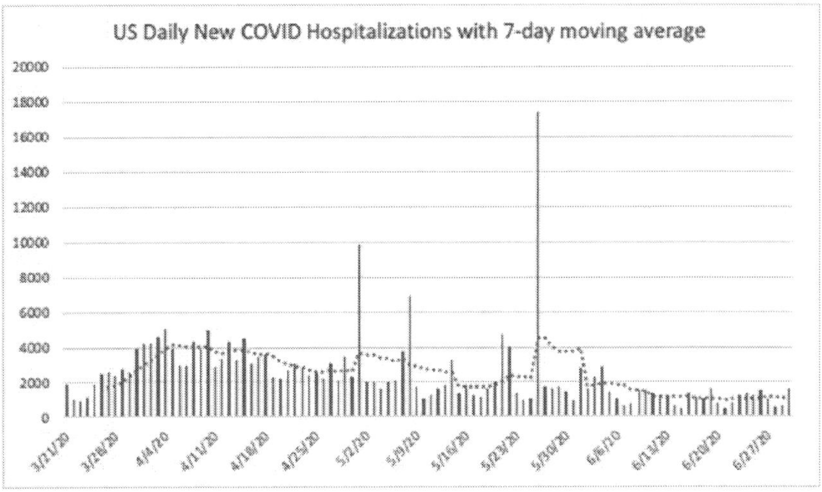


So what do these trends mean? How can the number of people currently hospitalized for COVID be rising while the number of new hospitalizations stays relatively low?

One answer is that hospital stays must be getting longer. If the increase in cases is picking up how infection is spreading, then the hospitalization data can help us see how serious those cases are. Looking at the ratio of new hospitalizations to new cases suggests that fewer of those infected need to be hospitalized.

The chart below indicates that the ratio of hospitalizations to infections is roughly a quarter of what it was in mid-April. This presents an even more complex puzzle: More people are currently in the hospital with COVID, but new hospitalizations are relatively low with a flat trend over the past few weeks. And on top of that, a smaller portion of those infected need to be hospitalized. And deaths continue to fall. The virus appears to be spreading as quickly as ever, but with fewer new hospitalizations and deaths, and longer hospital stays.

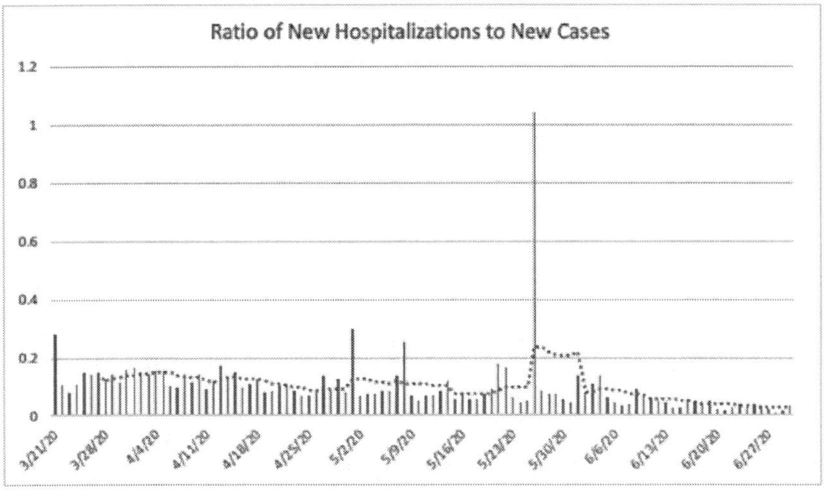


To understand how that may be happening, we need to disaggregate the data a bit, and examine how the trends in hospitalizations differ across the states.

## COMPARING HOSPITALIZATIONS AT THE STATE LEVEL

The table below uses four basic categories of states based on their hospitalization data and based on where their current numbers are relative to mid-April: Increasing trend, decreasing trend, flat trend, and insufficient data.

Currently 14 states have increasing trends, several of which were showing flat trends a few weeks ago. 24 states and the District of Columbia show clear downward trends, and eight have essentially flat trends. Of those eight, some could be categorized as increasing, but in those cases the number of hospitalizations have stayed low (often in or near the single digits) such that they could be considered "flat near zero."

Montana, for example, had 21 COVID hospitalizations on April 15th and currently has 12. On May 15 Montana had 3 COVID hospitalizations. The numbers are so small that no trend is identifiable. The same is true for Alaska, North Dakota, and Wyoming.

| STATES WITH INCREASED HOSPITALIZATIONS SINCE MID-APRIL | STATES (INCLUDING D.C.) WITH DECREASED HOSPITAL-IZATIONS SINCE MID-APRIL | STATES WITH FLAT HOSPITALIZATION TRENDS | STATES WITH INSUFFICIENT DATA |
|---|---|---|---|
| 1. Alabama | 1. Colorado | 1. Nebraska | 1. Florida |
| 2. Arkansas | 2. Connecticut | 2. North Dakota | 2. Hawaii |
| 3. Arizona | 3. D.C. | 3. Montana | 3. Idaho |
| 4. California | 4. Delaware | 4. Alaska | 4. Kansas |
| 5. Georgia | 5. Iowa | 5. New Mexico | |
| 6. Kentucky | 6. Illinois | 6. Oklahoma | |
| 7. Minnesota | 7. Indiana | 7. South Dakota | |
| 8. Mississippi | 8. Louisiana | 8. Wyoming | |
| 9. North Carolina | 9. Massachusetts | | |
| 10. Nevada | 10. Maryland | | |
| 11. South Carolina | 11. Maine | | |
| 12. Tennessee | 12. Michigan | | |
| 13. Texas | 13. Missouri | | |
| 14. Utah | 14. New Hampshire | | |
| | 15. New Jersey | | |
| | 16. New York | | |
| | 17. Ohio | | |
| | 18. Oregon | | |
| | 19. Pennsylvania | | |
| | 20. Rhode Island | | |
| | 21. Virginia | | |
| | 22. Vermont | | |
| | 23. Washington | | |
| | 24. Wisconsin | | |
| | 25. West Virginia | | |

Among the states with increasing trends, the current and new hospitalization data are sometimes contradictory. As of June 30, Alabama had 776 current hospitalizations, which is certainly more than that figure likely was in mid-April or even mid-May; the current hospitalizations do not go back that far for Alabama. The level of new hospitalizations has been around 30 per day since April. The seven-day average is slightly higher than it was a week ago, but roughly the same as it was a little over two weeks ago.

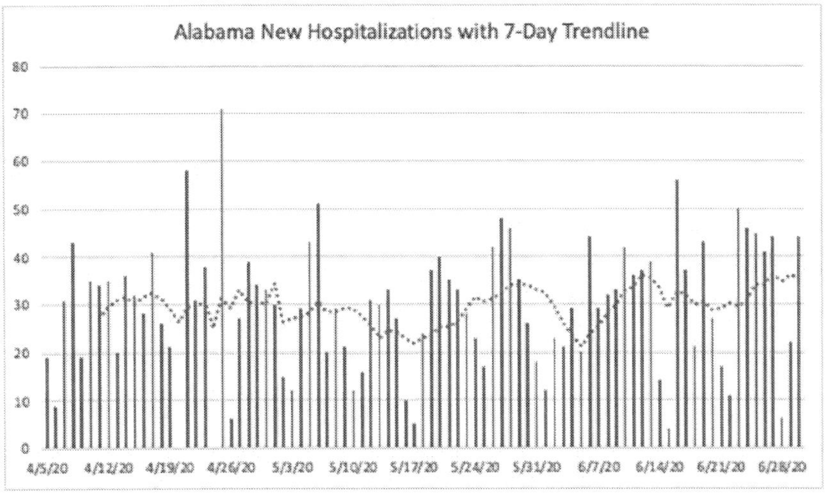


Georgia's current hospitalization goes back a bit farther than Alabama's, but not back to mid-April. Because of Georgia's steady increase in current hospitalizations for the past two weeks, it seems likely that its current hospitalizations are higher than they were ten weeks ago. Similar to Alabama, new hospitalizations seem relatively flat, near their levels in both mid-May and slightly lower than their levels in mid-April.

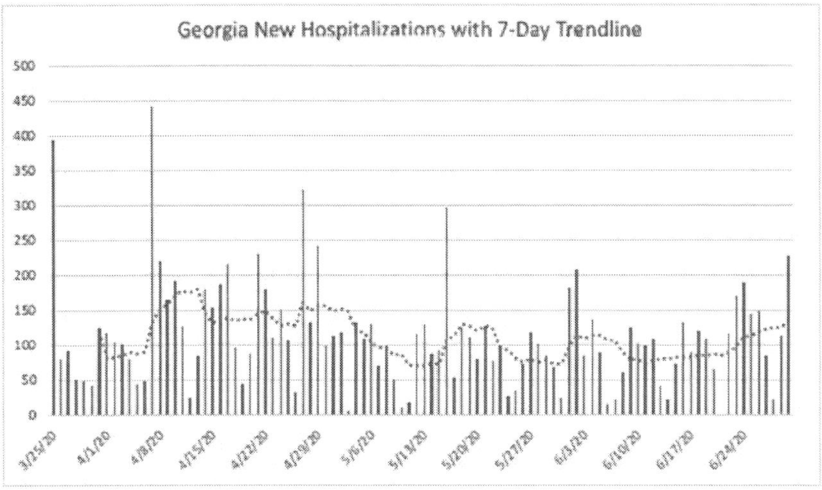

Other states have clear upward trends, such as North Carolina. But it is important to keep the magnitudes on the vertical axes of these charts in mind. North Carolina's current hospitalizations, below, give the impression of a strong upward trend. The next chart puts that trend in perspective, by comparing hospitalizations in North Carolina (population of 10.5 million) to those of New Jersey (population of 8.9 million).

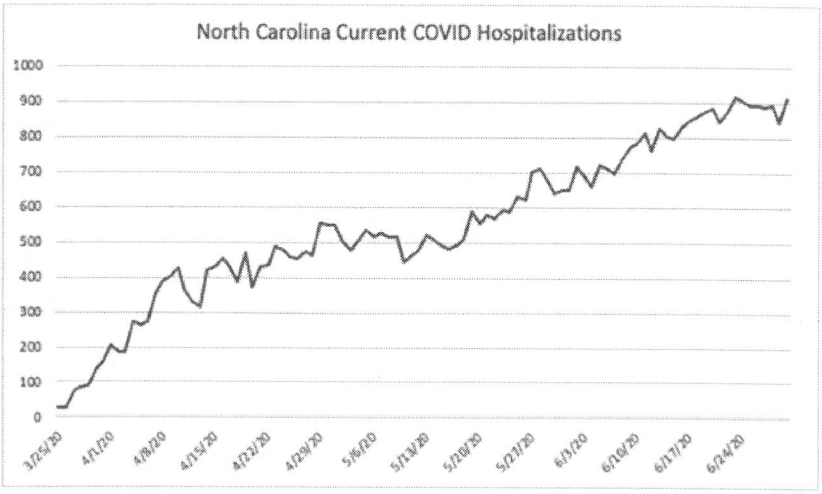


While the above chart suggests a sharp increase in hospitalizations, the comparison to New Jersey below makes North Carolina's increase appear gradual, as though they have successfully "flattened the curve."

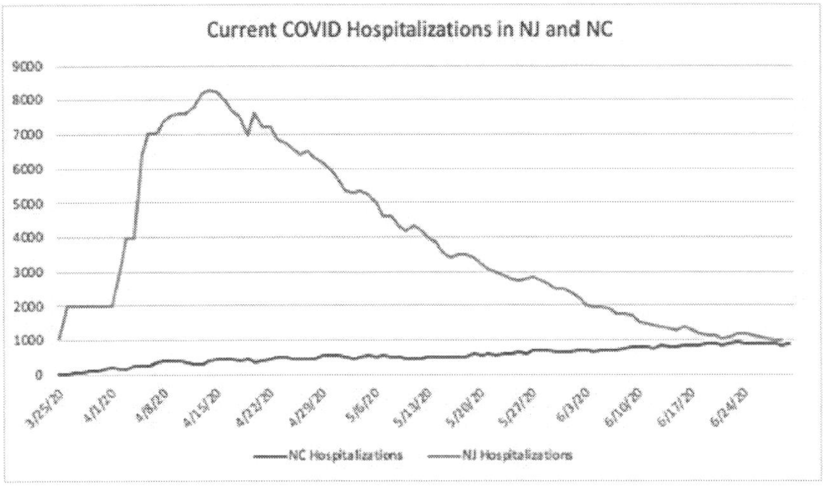


A similar comparison can be made between Texas (population of 29 million) and New York State (population of 19.5 million):

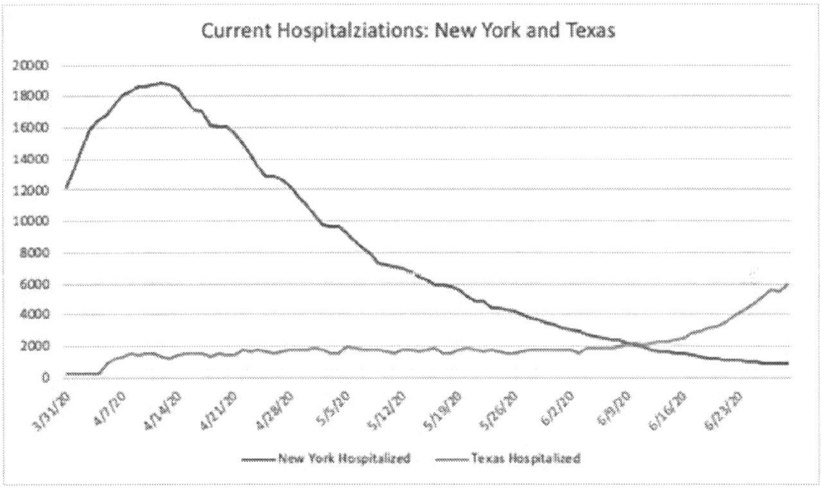


Despite the rapid increase in hospitalizations in Texas and its 30 percent larger population, it currently has a third of the people hospitalized today as New York did in mid-April. The trend in Texas is concerning, and worth watching closely. The reason to watch the trend is to guard against overwhelming the health care system's capacity. Surely New York came very close to doing just that, but it seems unlikely that Texas is close to exceeding its available resources at the moment.

Arizona has seen an increase in the past few weeks that is comparable to Texas. When compared to Northeastern states, Arizona's population of 7.3 million is closest to Massachusetts at 6.9 million. Given its trend, Arizona may well see hospitalization numbers similar to Massachusetts.

At the moment, though, it has roughly 1,000 fewer current hospitalizations than Massachusetts did at its peak. Similar to Texas, public health officials should monitor current hospitalizations as they consider ways to temporarily increase their capacity for treatment.

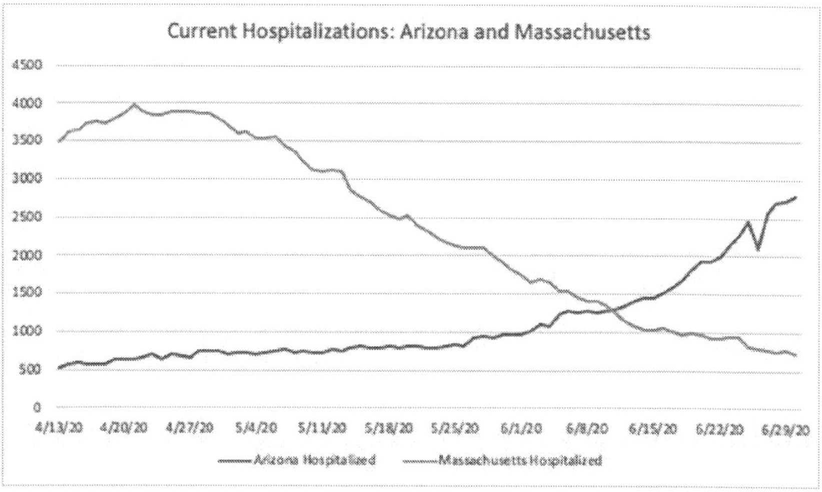


According to the COVID Tracking Project (CTP), 4 states do not report current hospitalizations. California, on the other hand, does not report cumulative hospitalization numbers to the CTP. Nonetheless, we know that California's current trend, despite its much larger population of 39.5 million, is very gradual compared with New York's. Comparing their current hospitalizations suggests that California has "flattened the curve" despite its large population and major metropolitan centers.

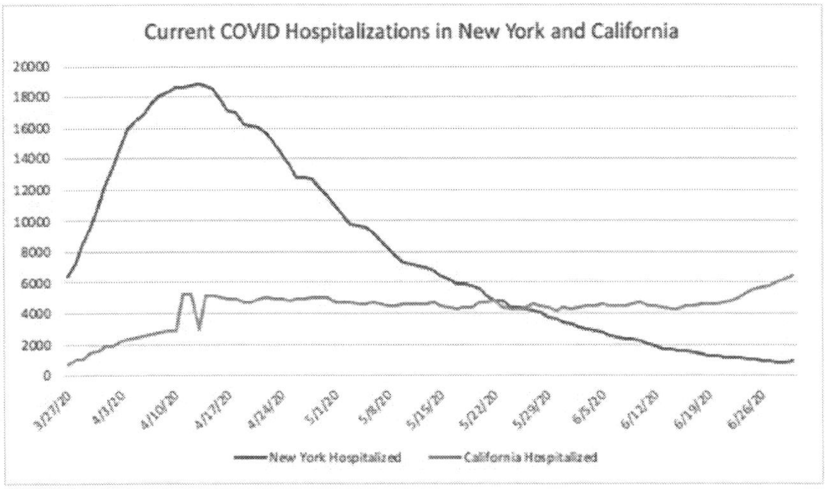


Florida, as one of the four states without current hospitalization numbers, can only be compared to other states on the basis of daily new hospitalizations. Florida's population, at 21.5 million, is 10 percent larger than New York's. Similar to other states currently seeing an increase in cases, the overall trend is much flatter than states with slightly smaller populations in the Northeast.

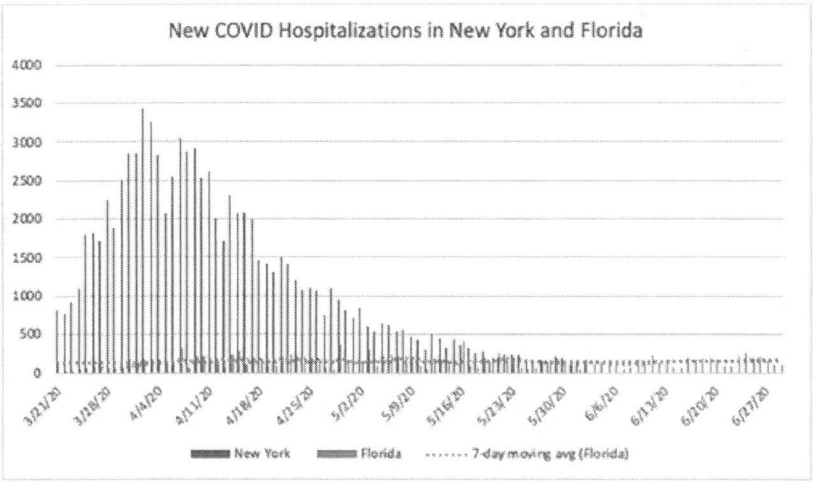

In all of the states that have seen an increase in hospitalizations since April, the absolute numbers are much smaller than states with similar (or in some cases much smaller) populations. More importantly, the trends are flatter, generally with more gradual increases over a much longer period of time, which is precisely what stay-at-home orders and school and business closures were intended to accomplish.

I focused on hospitalizations because they are the most relevant measure when it comes to the stated goals of preventative measures, i.e. to "flatten the curve." The objective behind prevention is to slow the spread of the virus, so that our health care providers and facilities would not be overwhelmed.

However, the data on COVID deaths are an important consideration. Deaths in most states with growing case numbers are still relatively flat. Similar to the hospitalization numbers, the absolute numbers are much lower in the South and Southeast than they were in the Northeast. In fact, the deaths are quite a bit lower in some cases. New York currently has very low death numbers, but they are similar to Florida's as seen below.

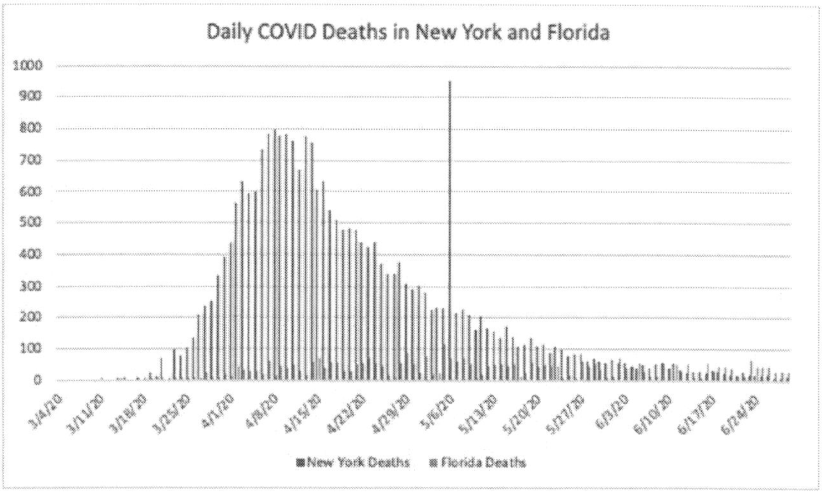

Overall, to the extent that people in the South and Southeast appear to not be taking COVID's spread as seriously as people in the Northeast, it is because the pandemic is not as serious in those states. The absolute numbers of hospitalizations and deaths are much lower, and the spread of the virus has been much slower.

## DEBATING DIFFERENCES

An obvious response to the comparisons above is to note that while New York, New Jersey, Massachusetts, and other Northeastern states may be comparable to Florida, North Carolina, Georgia, Arizona, and Texas in terms of population, they are much different in other ways. New York obviously has a much greater population density than Texas or Florida.

That is the point of making the comparisons, to highlight the fact that these differences matter when it comes to COVID's impact. Population density, demographics, and a number of other differences have slowed the spread and lessened the virus's impact on those states. It cannot be argued that the policy response has been more strict in those states or that the residents have been more vigilant.

Some may speculate that warmer weather or higher Vitamin D levels are part of the story. What is obvious is that states in the South have characteristics that make it harder for COVID to spread. It may just be the luck of having had exposure to similar viruses that enhance their residents' immune response to the virus.[141] It may be that by the time the virus started to spread quickly in these areas that it has evolved to become less deadly. Those are medical research questions

---

141 Leslie, Mitch. 2020. "T cells found in coronavirus patients 'bode well' for long-term immunity." *Science*, 368(6493): 809-810.

to be settled later.

What we can see clearly from the trends around the world is that the virus's impact has been very uneven, and massive outbreaks like those experienced in Italy and New York are not inevitable, and seem to have little to do with how local government addressed the pandemic. The states discussed above have all eased restrictions to different degrees on different timelines, yet the ones with the strictest policies are not systematically better off than those with the least restrictions.

So what about the puzzle of how current hospitalizations can increase while new hospitalizations remain flat and deaths continue to decline? As Peter C. Earle pointed out, infections have tended to grow more quickly among younger people recently.[142] Many of those young people still seek treatment, although their symptoms are less severe than they tend to be for older patients. And we know that medical facilities have an incentive to increase their counts of COVID hospitalizations.[143]

Since the virus is far less deadly among younger people, even when large numbers are infected deaths can continue to fall. Those who are hospitalized are more likely to live, which combined with better treatment protocols can increase the number of people living in the hospital at a given point in time. As more of those people recover, the virus's impact is lessened even further.

---

142 See article herein entitled "The Real Pandemic Was a Nursing Home Problem." *American Institute for Economic Research*, June 30.

143 Stringham, Edward Peter. 2020. "Why We Should Not Be Concerned About Increasing Covid-19 Cases in Texas." *American Institute for Economic Research*, July 2.

## TWO PANDEMICS: ONE SERIOUS, ONE MILD

BY PHILLIP W. MAGNESS

July 3, 2020

Epidemiological modeling has played a central role in the global response to the novel coronavirus (COVID-19) outbreak of early 2020. The response to the emerging pandemic prompted multiple teams of researchers to rapidly adapt existing models, predominantly from previous influenza outbreaks, to forecast the spread of COVID-19 as well as its anticipated fatality rates.

Using the familiar SIR/SEIR epidemiology models, these studies attempt to employ modern statistical techniques to predict the spread and expected mortality of the COVID-19 pandemic.[144] Common approaches include mechanistic adaptations of agent-based simulation to the SIR/SEIR framework that probabilistically estimate the spread of the virus through general social interactions, as well as autoregressive forecasting techniques that update to reflect emerging data for the disease's spread in a specific country or locale. In both cases, the associated models have been used to strongly advise the adoption of non-pharmaceutical policy interventions as a primary tool of COVID-19 mitigation.[145]

These interventions, consisting of the now-familiar suite of public event cancellations, school and business closures, and wide scale lockdowns or shelter-in-place orders (SIPOs), were implemented in all but a handful of countries across the globe—often with direct

---

144 Wikipedia. 2020. "Compartmental models in epidemiology." *Wikipedia*, July 22.

145 Landler and Castle (2020); Adam (2020).

dependence on the advice of epidemiology modeling. In a well-documented example, the influential simulation model for the United Kingdom and the United States by researchers at Imperial College London (ICL) spurred both governments to shift their response strategies to embrace wide scale lockdowns in mid-March 2020.[146]

American President Donald Trump and UK Prime Minister Boris Johnson directly credited this model for their respective decisions to impose lockdowns, and Trump continues to cite the ICL projections of up to 2.2 million deaths to justify his actions. These fantastical claims increasingly diverge from the realities of the coronavirus outbreak. In the time since its release back in March, the ICL model has repeatedly failed to accurately anticipate the course of the pandemic in both countries, and in its adaptation to other locales such as Sweden.[147]

While most of the policy discussion has thus far focused on society-wide interventions aimed at reducing the spread of COVID-19 in the general population, the problem of acute outbreaks within long-term care facilities (LTCs) such as nursing homes is now difficult to deny.[148] Although LTC outbreak data vary widely in scope and quality by state and country, a high concentration of COVID-related deaths in such facilities is readily apparent. Depending on jurisdiction, it is not uncommon to find between 30 and 70 percent of recorded COVID-19 fatalities have occurred in nursing homes, including more than half of all

---

146 Ferguson et al. (2020).

147 See article herein entitled "SimCity-Style Modeling Flunks the Real-World Test"; Magness, Phillip W. 2020. "Imperial College Model Applied to Sweden Yields Preposterous Results." *American Institute for Economic Research,* April 30.

148 See article herein entitled "The Real Pandemic Was a Nursing Home Problem."

recorded deaths in Europe. Similar patterns appear in most US states.[149]

The concentration of outbreaks in LTCs has only recently called attention to a shortcoming of the epidemiological modeling approach that guided the world's COVID-19 response strategies. While these models aim to project the disease's spread through social interactions within the general population, they do not appear to be suitable for capturing acute outbreaks among susceptible populations in LTCs and similar closed-residential facilities.[150]

Indeed, we may find this shortcoming directly acknowledged in the 2006 influenza pandemic study that the Imperial College team used as the basis of their COVID-19 simulation.[151] As its authors conceded at the time, "[l]ack of data prevent us from reliably modelling transmission in the important contexts of residential institutions (for example, care homes, prisons) and health care settings."

The conundrum presented by LTC outbreaks vis-à-vis epidemiological modeling need not be speculative though, as emerging statistical patterns are beginning to reveal a sharp divergence in the pandemic's course when trends in such facilities are compared to the general population. Although LTC outbreaks have accounted for significant shares of COVID-19 mortality in all 50 states, obtaining accurate and daily LTC data remains a challenge.

The Commonwealth of Massachusetts presents an exception to this

---

149 2020. "Nursing Home/LTC COVID Deaths By State." *GoogleSheet.*

150 Pillemer, Karl, Lakshminarayana Subramanian, and Nathaniel Hupert. 2020. "The Importance of Long-term Care Populations in Models of COVID-19." *JAMA*, 324(1): 25-26.

151 Ferguson, Neil M., Derek A.T. Cummings, Christophe Fraser, James C. Cajka, Philip C. Cooley, and Donald S. Burke. 2006. "Strategies for mitigating an influenza pandemic." *Nature*, April 26.

data deficit.[152] Ranking among the hardest-hit of US states outside of the New York City region, Massachusetts began tracking detailed daily COVID-19 case and mortality statistics for LTC facilities on April 10, 2020. At this relatively early stage in the pandemic, LTC and non-LTC fatalities in Massachusetts sat at near-parity. They then began to rapidly diverge. As of June 29, LTC deaths account for 5,111 out of 7,895 confirmed deaths in the commonwealth, or 64.7 percent of all fatalities.

The clear patterns in these data suggest that the coronavirus would be better understood if we began to treat it as two simultaneous pandemics: one severe but acute outbreak that ravages nursing homes and LTCs with extremely high fatalities concentrated among the elderly and infirm, and a second significantly milder wave in the general population.

As nearly all mitigation strategies have focused on containing the spread in the general population through lockdowns and similar mandates, the policy response has almost entirely missed the mark despite unleashing unprecedented devastation to our economy and social fabric.

Daily data from Massachusetts illustrate the divergence of the two simultaneous pandemics. As may be seen in the chart below, they show steady growth in the share of COVID-19 deaths arising from LTC facility outbreaks since the beginning of record keeping. Furthermore, these two trends continue to split apart. For the month of June, Massachusetts averaged only 9 COVID-19 deaths per day in the general population. By contrast, the state's LTC facilities averaged 27 deaths per day despite comprising a tiny share of the population.

---

152 Mass.Gov. 2020. "Archive of COVID-19 cases in Massachusetts." *Mass.gov.*

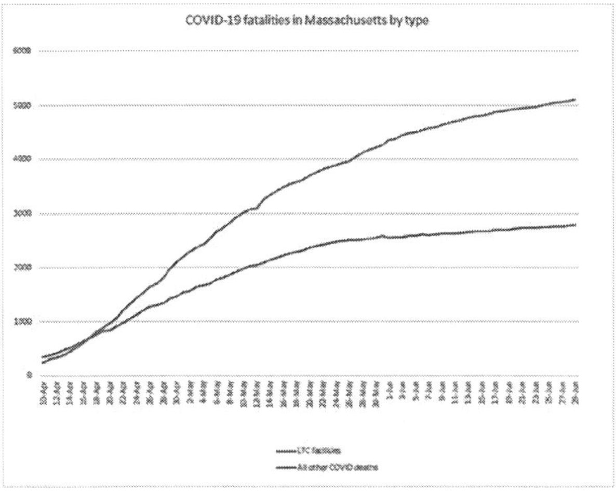


When smoothed using a 7-day moving average, daily deaths in the non-LTC general population peaked in late April and began to sharply decline in late May 2020. While Massachusetts LTC deaths have leveled from their early peak around the same time, they still remain at approximately three times the general population's daily toll.

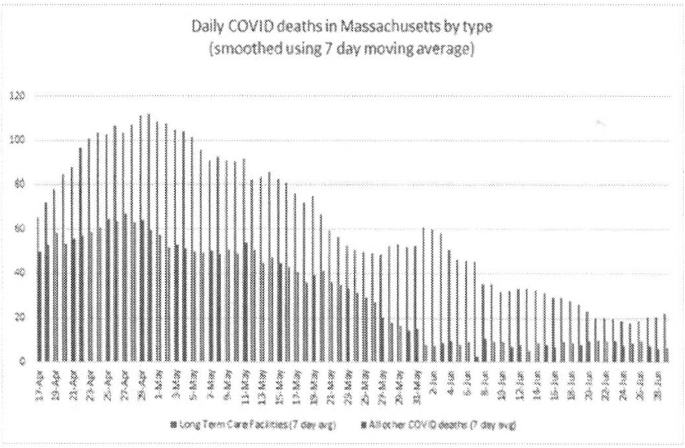


*Note: Massachusetts changed its counting methodology on June 1 to include probable COVID-19 deaths that were not confirmed by direct testing. The brief spike in LTC deaths from around this time is likely an artifact of this change in reporting, and not the brief spike observed in the chart.*

The severity of the LTC outbreak may be seen in the cumulative death toll from this subset of the population. As of this writing, COVID-19 mortalities appear to encompass almost 10 percent of the commonwealth's pre-pandemic LTC population of an estimated 53,000 residents. By comparison, the state's approximately 2,784 non-LTC general population deaths as of June 30th come from an estimated 6.9 million people.

The clear difference between observed patterns in LTCs and the general population points to a need to further assess the suitability of current COVID-19 epidemiological modeling strategies in accurately capturing the dynamics of the ongoing pandemic. Indeed, the modeling approach appears to project an entirely different mortality pattern than what we are observing in realized data—even when cumulative death totals approximate some of the milder modeled scenarios from the ICL model and similar projections.

Since most policy interventions aimed at mitigating COVID-19 were premised upon models depicting its general population spread, the emerging evidence of a very different pattern concentrated in LTC facilities is of high consequence in evaluating the political interventions adopted back in March.

Simply put, we adopted the wrong measures and used them to ineffectually target the milder of the two pandemics, all the while neglecting or even exacerbating the much more severe outbreak that continues to run its course through our vulnerable nursing home population.[153]

---

153 Condon, Bernard, Jennifer Peltz, and Jim Mustian. 2020. "AP count: Over 4,500 virus patients sent to NY nursing homes." *ABC News*, May 22.

# POWER AND ERROR

## PROFESSOR LOCKDOWN NOW CLAIMS TO HAVE SAVED 3.1 MILLION LIVES

BY PHILLIP W. MAGNESS

June 9, 2020

The problem of causal inference presents one of the great challenges of empirical analysis. While it is relatively easy to find patterns in data that appear to move over time in response to overlapping events, it is much harder to show that those events specifically *caused* the data to move as expected.

Think about how presidents often cite positive economic data such as GDP growth or the stock market as vindication of their own economic policies. Prior to early March 2020 this was a favorite tweeting topic of Donald Trump, although his predecessors almost all made similar claims. While this argument makes for a useful campaign pitch, it is poor social science and would never pass empirical scrutiny.

To solve the causal inference problem, social scientists usually enlist sophisticated statistical tools that are designed to isolate the effects of a known event on a data trend or pattern by comparing it to an independent or unaffected counterfactual. With rigorous testing and good data, they may *infer* causality by comparison with natural experiments, usually involving ruling out a series of alternative explanations.

To use a concrete example, consider the ongoing question about the effectiveness of the COVID-19 lockdown policies employed in several U.S. states as well as other countries. A causal inference test of the lockdowns would require clear evidence of different outcomes between states that adopted shelter-in-place rules and states that did not. Given the complex multitude of confounding variables affecting COVID-19 transmission and mortality rates, isolating causality from the lockdown policies is no easy task.

That brings us to a new report published in the journal *Nature* by the epidemiology team at Imperial College-London (ICL), including Neil Ferguson of some fame.[154] This is the same epidemiology research center whose agent-based simulation model convinced the American and British governments to switch to a lockdown strategy.[155]

The study purports to demonstrate "that major non-pharmaceutical interventions and lockdown in particular have had a large effect on reducing transmission" of the COVID-19 virus. The paper and an accompanying press release from the university put numbers to this claim, asserting that the lockdowns saved an estimated 3.1 million lives in Europe.[156]

Although this headline-grabbing claim will likely be treated as a vindication of the lockdown approach by its political supporters, a closer look at the analysis suggests the Imperial College team reached this conclusion without offering a viable causal inference strategy. As they describe in the paper, "By comparing the deaths predicted under the model with no interventions to the deaths predicted in our intervention model, we calculated the total deaths averted in our study period."

Put differently, the epidemiologists reached their estimates by taking the difference between observed deaths and their own agent-based simulation of COVID interventions, including the lockdowns. They

---

154 Glaxman, Seth, Swapnil Mishra, Axel Gandy, H. Juliette T. Unwin, Thomas A. Mellan et al. 2020. "Estimating the effects of non-pharmaceutical interventions on COVID-19 in Europe." *Nature*, June 8.

155 See article herein entitled "SimCity-Style Modeling Flunks the Real-World Test"; Landler, Mark, and Stephen Castle. 2020. "Behind the Virus Report That Jarred the U.S. and the U.K. to Action." *The New York Times*, April 2.

156 Wighton, Kate. 2020. "Lockdown and school closures in Europe may have prevented 3.1m deaths." *Imperial College London*, June 8.

then depict the difference as if it demonstrates the validity of their own simulation model, despite providing no evidence that their original simulation was correct.

Table 1 from the study shows this basic arithmetic exercise across 11 different European countries:

**Forecasted deaths since the beginning of the epidemic up to 4th May in our model vs. a counterfactual model assuming no interventions had taken place**

| Country | Observed Deaths up to 4th May<br>(observed) | Model estimated deaths up to 4th May<br>(our model) | Model estimated deaths up to 4th May<br>(counterfactual model assuming no interventions have occurred) | Model deaths averted up to 4th May<br>(difference between counterfactual and actual) |
|---|---|---|---|---|
| Austria | 600 | 620 [520 - 720] | 66,000 [40,000 - 86,000] | 65,000 [40,000 - 85,000] |
| Belgium | 7,924 | 7,300 [6,400 - 8,400] | 120,000 [93,000 – 140,000] | 110,000 [86,000 – 130,000] |
| Denmark | 493 | 500 [430 - 590] | 34,000 [17,000 - 50,000] | 34,000 [17,000 - 49,000] |
| France | 25,201 | 23,000 [21,000 - 27,000] | 720,000 [590,000 - 850,000] | 690,000 [570,000 - 820,000] |
| Germany | 6,831 | 6,800 [6,000 - 7,900] | 570,000 [370,000 - 780,000] | 560,000 [370,000 - 770,000] |
| Italy | 29,079 | 31,000 [27,000 - 35,000] | 670,000 [540,000 - 800,000] | 630,000 [510,000 - 760,000] |
| Norway | 208 | 210 [170 - 250] | 12,000 [3,400 - 24,000] | 12,000 [3,200 - 23,000] |
| Spain | 25,613 | 25,000 [22,000 - 28,000] | 470,000 [390,000 - 560,000] | 450,000 [360,000 – 540,000] |
| Sweden | 2,769 | 2,800 [2,500 - 3,300] | 28,000 [15,000 - 49,000] | 26,000 [12,000 - 46,000] |
| Switzerland | 1,476 | 1,500 [1,300 - 1,800] | 54,000 [36,000 - 73,000] | 52,000 [34,000 - 71,000] |
| United Kingdom | 28,734 | 29,000 [25,000 - 34,000] | 500,000 [400,000 - 610,000] | 470,000 [370,000 – 580,000] |
| All | 128,928 | 130,000<br>[120,000 - 140,000] | 3,200,000<br>[2,900,000 - 3,600,000] | 3,100,000<br>[2,800,000 - 3,500,000] |

The problem with this approach is that it attempts to imply causality by attributing the observed death tolls to the effectiveness of the lockdowns, which they then claim to demonstrate through nothing more than a self-referential appeal to their own simulation model for a "no intervention" counterfactual.

If that line of argument sounds familiar, it's because Donald Trump beat the Imperial College team to the punch. Citing the now-infamous March 16$^{th}$ ICL report by Imperial's Neil Ferguson, the American president now regularly claims vindication for his own support of the lockdowns on account of the difference between its 2 million-plus projected death toll and the actual count of just over 100,000 as of this writing.[157]

As Trump tweeted on May 26,

> For all of the political hacks out there, if I hadn't done my job well, & early, we would have lost 1 1/2 to 2 Million People, as opposed to the 100,000 plus that looks like will be the number.[158]

Whether used by Imperial College or Trump, this line of argument falters as social science because it assumes the validity of the very same forecast it purports to demonstrate. Rather than testing the causal inference that lockdowns reduced the COVID death rate, it takes their own forecasted death rate as a given and then purports to calculate the number of lives saved by simple subtraction from its own model.

That approach only works if one begins from the assumption that the Imperial College's "no intervention" model is axiomatically true. The new paper essentially acknowledges as much in noting that "the counterfactual model without interventions is illustrative only and reflects our model assumptions." Rather than investigating this seemingly-crucial assertion further, let alone subjecting it to empirical testing, the

---

157 Ferguson, Neil M., Daniel Laydon, Gemma Nedjati-Gilani, Natsuko Imai, Kylie Ainslie et al. 2020. "Impact of non-pharmaceutical interventions (NPIs) to reduce COVID-19 mortality and healthcare demand." *Imperial College COVID-19 Response Team*, Report No. 9.

158 Trump, Donald J. (@realDonaldTrump). 2020. "For all of the political hacks out there, if I hadn't done my job well, & early, we would have lost 1 1/2 to 2 Million People, as opposed to the 100,000 plus that looks like will be the number[...]" *Twitter*, May 26, 2020.

authors indulge in a handwaving exercise that simply declares: "Given this agreement in differing scenarios we believe our estimates for the counterfactual deaths averted to be plausible."

This conclusion is rendered untenable by the many already-documented flaws in the original ICL model. That model failed to account for the effects of human behavioral modification on its results.[159] It neglected to run robustness checks on its own assumptions about the effectiveness of lockdowns. It resulted in preposterously unrealistic death toll projections when applied to Sweden, which eschewed lockdowns for a lighter-touch policy.[160] And there is even evidence that the ICL model design has no means of accounting for nursing home transmission of the disease—the largest single factor in COVID-related deaths.[161]

These and other findings provide several reasons to doubt the main causal mechanism of the ICL model, linking lockdowns to sizable claims about the reduction of COVID fatalities.

The result is not a valid exercise in social scientific analysis, nor is it even an empirically robust test of the ICL model's performance. Like Trump's tweeting about both the economy before March 2020 and his own claimed role in reducing COVID deaths after the lockdowns, it is an exercise in statistical astrology.

Sadly, unlike Trump's tweets, however, the ICL managed to convince *Nature*, a top journal in the profession, to publish these unfounded claims.

---

159 Magness, Phillip W. 2020. "How Wrong Were the Models and Why?" *American Institute for Economic Research*, April 23.

160 Magness, Phillip W. 2020. "Imperial College Model Applied to Sweden Yields Preposterous Results." *American Institute for Economic Research*, April 30.

161 See article herein entitled "SimCity-style Modeling Flunks the Real-World Test."

## WHAT ECONOMISTS CAN TEACH EPIDEMIOLOGISTS

BY PETER C. EARLE

July 11, 2020

As data accrues on both a national and state-by-state basis, the parameters of COVID-19's lethality is firming up. Two new papers from Dr. John Ioannidis point to the growing shortfall between apocalyptic pandemic predictions and the vastly more destructive policies implemented in observance of them.[162]

The first, entitled "Population-level COVID-19 mortality risk for non-elderly individuals overall and for non-elderly individuals without underlying diseases in pandemic epicenters" offers more evidence supporting the assertion that the government reaction to the virus has been vastly overwrought.[163]

Using data from 11 European countries, 12 US states, and Canada, Ioannidis and his team show that the infection rate is much higher than previously thought, which suggests that both the incidence of asymptomatic and mildly symptomatic cases is higher than thought, and the fatality rate much lower than previously estimated.

As regards the age of victims,

---

162 Stringham, Edward Peter. 2020. "Who Is John Ioannidis?" *American Institute for Economic Research*, April 19.

163 Ioannidis, John P.A., Catherine Axfors, and Despina G. Contopoulos-Ioannidis. 2020. "Population-level COVID-19 mortality risk for non-elderly individuals overall and for nonelderly individuals without underlying diseases in pandemic epicenters." *medRxiv.*

> People [under] 65 years old have very small risks of COVID-19 death even in pandemic epicenters and deaths for people [under] 65 years without underlying predisposing conditions are remarkably uncommon. Strategies focusing specifically on protecting high-risk elderly individuals should be considered in managing the pandemic.

In the other paper, "Forecasting for COVID-19 has failed," Ioanndis and co-authors take aim at the reasons for which the predictions were so incredibly inaccurate.[164] Early predictions included that New York needed up to 140,000 hospital beds for stricken COVID-19 victims; the total number of individuals hospitalized was 18,569.

In California on March 17, 2020, it was predicted that "at least 1.2 million people over the age of 18 [would] need hospitalization from the disease," which would require 50,000 additional hospital beds. In fact, "COVID-19 patients [ultimately] occupied fewer than two in 10 beds."

On March 27, 2020, Vice Provost for Global Initiatives at the University of Pennsylvania, Ezekiel Emanuel predicted that there would 100,000,000 COVID-19 cases in the United States in the four subsequent weeks—slightly less than one in three of all Americans. Unsurprisingly, this prediction has since been taken down.[165]

---

164 Ioannidis, John P.A., Sally Cripps, and Martin A. Tanner. 2020. "Forecasting for COVID-19 has failed." *International Institute of Forecasters*, June 11.

165 N.d. "Ezekiel J. Emanuel." *Ezekiel J. Emanuel.*

www.realclearpolitics.com › video › 2020/03/27 › ezekiel...

Ezekiel Emanuel: U.S. Will Have 100 Million Cases Of COVID ...

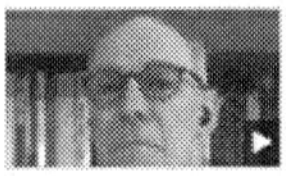

Ezekiel Emanuel: U.S. Will Have 100 Million Cases Of COVID-19 In Four Weeks, Doubling Every Four Days ...
Mar 27, 2020

Divination, accurate or not, is harmless in and of itself: that's obvious. But when made by scientific dignitaries, in particular in the process of informing politicians amid crisis circumstances, it often leads to knee jerk reactions at all levels. The causative factors cited are, or should be, well known to economists: they include use of poor data or the wrong use of high quality data; improper or incorrect assumptions; wrongful estimates of sensitivity; wrongly interpreted past results or evidence; problems of dimensionality; and groupthink/bandwagon effects.[166]

From a high level, epidemiological forecasts failed for the very reason that econometric predictions often flounder: the uncritical importation of modeling techniques from physics or applied mathematics into social science realms. This should not be especially revelatory. In *The Counter-Revolution of Science*, F. A. Hayek noted the pernicious effects of applying rigidly quantitative concepts where human action is at work, attributing them to "an ambition to imitate science in its methods rather than its spirit."[167]

Using Ioannidis' guidelines, a subset of the elements which lead to predictive failures in epidemiology can not only be examined, but analogized directly with economic and econometric counterparts.

---

166 AP. 2007. "Bernanke: Subprime Mortgage Woes Won't Seriously Hurt Economy." *CNBC*, May 17.

167 Hayek, F.A. 1952. *The Counter-Revolution of Science*. The Free Press: Glencoe, IL.

## DATA PROBLEMS

The issue of data quality and application in economics is one which arose from the growing quantification of the social sciences.[168] Data which is either erroneously recorded, speciously accurate, or completely fabricated has been a problem of legendary proportions in econometrics and in the crafting of economic policy.[169]

Although first identified as a serious issue 70 years ago, less than three years after the publication of the pivotal work, *Foundations of Economic Analysis* by Paul A. Samuelson, the mathematization of economics has proceeded apace with virtually no embracing of Oskar Morgenstern's cautions.[170]

Similarly, there is growing evidence that some COVID-19 related data has been problematic: erroneous or miscalculated.[171] Where testing is concerned, even a 1% error in the tens of millions of coronavirus tests being conducted would amount to hundreds of thousands of misdiagnoses, with the knock-on effects that such results give rise to.

---

168 Weintraub, E. Roy. 2002. *How Economics Became a Mathematical Science.* Duke University Press: UK.

169 While not waxing conspiratorially, it bears mentioning that low-quality data can be as much a political tool as a source of imprecision in both epidemiology and economics.

170 Morgenstern (1963); Samuelson, Paul A. 1947. *Foundations of Economic Analysis.* Harvard University Press: US; Bagus, Philipp. 2011. "Morgenstern's Forgotten Contribution: A Stab to the Heart of Modern Economics." *The American Journal of Economics and Sociology*, April 14.

171 Steinbuch, Yaron. 2020. "Georgia Department of Health slammed for misleading coronavirus data." *New York Post*, May 19.

## ERRONEOUS ASSUMPTIONS

Untenable and oversimplifying assumptions in economic formulations are often defended as pragmatic or unavoidable.[172] These are problematic even when methodologies are appropriate, the data sound, and the calculations correct:

> Many [epidemiological] models assume homogeneity, i.e.all people having equal chances of mixing with each other and infecting each other. This is an untenable assumption and in reality, tremendous heterogeneity of exposures and mixing is likely to be the norm. Unless this heterogeneity is recognized, estimates of the proportion of people eventually infected before reaching her immunity can be markedly inflated.[173]

Epidemiologically, the homogeneity oversight is seen at its starkest and most tragically in comparing the outcome of insufficiently protecting the most vulnerable populations while simultaneously closing schools and excoriating teenagers/college students—among the least affected groups—for their social inclinations.[174]

---

172 Ivarola, Leonardo. 2018. "A plea for realistic assumptions in economic modelling." *Theoria: An International Journal for Theory, History and Foundations of Science*, 33(3): 417-433.

173 Ioannidis, Cripps and Tanner (2020).

174 See articles herein entitled "The Real Pandemic Was a Nursing Home Problem" and "Why Did they Close the Schools?"; Tucker, Jeffrey A. 2020. "The 2007 Origins of Forced School Closings and Mandatory Human Separation." *American Institute for Economic Research*, May 26; Associated Press. 2020. "Coronavirus: Cuomo upset with 'arrogant' New Yorkers who aren't social distancing." *Syracuse.com*, March 22.

## SENSITIVITY OF ESTIMATES

Determining how an independent variable or groups of independent variables affect dependent variables is the focus of sensitivity analysis. Depending upon the regression (or other operation) being performed, and in particular the presence of exponents, a small error in independent factors can lead to huge variances in outcomes.[175]

There are techniques which can be used to determine where, when, and to what degree estimates have a disproportionate impact on the outcome of simulations or calculations, whether that comes in the form of wildly overblown or unrealistically diminished outcomes. Often, though, sensitivity is seen not in models, but in the real world events they are designed to approximate.

Ioannidis cited the "inherent impossibility" of fixing such models, as the ubiquity of models employing "exponentiated variables [lead to] small errors [that] result in major deviations from reality." Morgenstern evinced similar concerns in 1950 regarding the curve-fitting propensities of the new wave of economic practice; here in production functions, but the criticism is certainly extendable:

> Consider, for example, the important problem of whether linear or nonlinear production functions should be considered in economic models. Non-linearity is a great complication and is, therefore, best avoided as much as possible. True non-linearity in the strict mathematical sense is avoided in physics as far as possible. Even quantum mechanics is treated as linear on

175 This is one of the characteristics of a chaotic system: the so-called butterfly effect refers to systems where ultimate outcomes or states show a tremendous degree of sensitivity to initial conditions.

> a higher level. Many apparently nonlinear phenomena, upon closer investigation, can well be treated as linear... The distinction is largely a matter of the precision of measurement, which is exactly where the weakness is strongest in economics. It is astonishing that economists seem to hesitate far less to introduce non-linearity than physical scientists, where the tradition of mathematical exploration is so much older and the experience with observation and measurement so much firmer.[176]

I would not deign to correct such a luminary as Dr. Morgenstern, but I would add that the weakness is not strongest in economics alone, but in all undertakings which quantitatively rigidify human action, whether individual or *en masse*.

## POOR PAST EVIDENCE ON EFFECTS OF AVAILABLE INTERVENTIONS

Unbeknownst to the vast majority of people who are or will suffer from the effects of the lockdowns, the "flatten-the-curve" efforts were informed by information from the Spanish Flu of 1918. Thus data of impeachable quality, from a pandemic event which occurred over one century ago, involving a different pathogen—as a major world war was ending, and when living conditions, longevity, the state of medical science, the tenor of social interactions, and countless other variables were immeasurably different—were applied to sculpt the government response to the outbreak of the novel coronavirus.

Ioannidis and his co-authors comment that "[w]hile some interventions... are likely to have beneficial effects, assuming huge benefits

176 Morgenstern (1963).

is incongruent with the past (weak) evidence and should be avoided. Large benefits may be feasible from precise, focused measures."[177] The idea that a single (or even a small handful) of studies might be used to buttress indefensible arguments or to support questionable plans is occasionally seen in economic policymaking as well.[178]

## DIMENSIONALITY

"Almost all models that had a prominent role in [pandemic] decision-making," Ioannidis continues, "focused on COVID-19 outcomes, often just a single outcome or a few outcomes (e.g., deaths or hospital needs). Models prime for decision making need to take into account the impact on multiple fronts (e.g. other aspects of healthcare, other diseases, dimensions of the economy, etc.)." Some remedies to this include interdisciplinary scrutiny of model outcomes and a look at past implementations in the face of pandemics—including those to which there was no response at all.

While dimensionality as a specific problem afflicts economic modeling as well, general comments in this regard closely echo the battered-but-unmoved screeds against one of the earliest fixtures of economic education: *ceteris paribus*, by which one considers causal

177 Ioannidis, Cripps, and Tanner (2020, p. 26).

178 Card, David, and Alan B. Krueger. 1993. "Minimum Wages and Employment: A Case Study of the Fast Food Industry in New Jersey and Pennsylvania." *NBER*, Working Paper No. 4509.

or empirical relations while holding other influences equal.[179] While a useful tool for educational purposes, when it creeps into crafting policies the results can be costly.[180]

## GROUPTHINK AND BANDWAGON EFFECTS

Ioannidis cites groupthink among epidemiologists as a source of forecasting error. When a doomsday prediction is made—especially by celebrity scientists—the act of introducing a more mitigating prognosis may bring substantial risk to one's career, and thus be suppressed. Alternatively, the published or broadcast results of thought leaders may be a form of anchoring. As Ioannidis and his team write,

> Models can be tuned to get desirable results and predictions, e.g. by changing the input of what are deemed to be the plausible values for key variables. This is true for models that depend upon theory and speculation, but even data-driven forecasting can do the same, depending upon how the modeling is performed. In the presence of strong groupthink and bandwagon effects, modelers may consciously fit their predictions to what the dominant thinking and expectations are—or they may be

---

179 At times, the *ceteris paribus* approach is defended by econometricians who liken it to the practice of ignoring air resistance in gravity experiments. It's a shamefully underhanded argument that immingles physical with social science phenomena.

Esteban-Bravo, Mercedes, and Francisco J. Nogales. 2005. "Reducing the curse of dimensionality in dynamic stochastic economic problems by decomposition methods."

180 Jhun, Jennifer S. 2016. "What's the Point of Ceteris Paribus? or, How to Understand Supply and Demand Curves." *Philosophy of Science*, 85(2): 271-292.

forced to do so.[181]

The economics profession is certainly not immune to this. It manifests in several ways, one of which is mainstream economists' unwillingness to admit their errors.[182] Many economists instinctively do not criticize theory or practices within their institution or school of thought owing to political expediency. The highly "siloed" nature of journals and conferences attests to it, as do the veritable echo chambers in social media. Cognitive and confirmation biases are noted as well.[183] These are not merely a personal observation; their effects have been cited elsewhere.[184] Here, in no less prominent a place as the International Monetary Fund:

> Analytical weaknesses were at the core of some of the IMF's most evident shortcomings in surveillance ... [as a result of] ... the tendency among homogeneous, cohesive groups to consider issues only within a certain paradigm and not challenge its basic premises.[185]

## THE MEDIA AMPLIFIER

Farcical predictions, whether owing to one or all of the above elements, would nevertheless be innocuous if limited to circulating among small

---

181 Ioannidis, Cripps, and Tanner (2020, p. 27).

182 As the continued use of flawed models or inexact numbers attests to.

183 Wikipedia. 2020. "Confirmation bias." *Wikipedia*, July 14.

184 IMF. 2011. "IMF Performance in the Run-Up to the Financial and Economic Crisis: IMF Surveillance in 2004-07." *International Monetary Fund*, August 24.

185 See Chapter 4 "Why Did the IMF Fail to Give Clear Warning?" in: IMF (2011).

groups of scientists or within the rarified pages of peer-reviewed journals. But whether viewed as a vital democratic institution, a propagandistic organ of political parties, or somewhere in between, it's far from a conspiracy theory to note that the dominant media outlets are massive businesses which fundamentally compete for revenue on the basis of attention. As with politicians, the loudest and scariest messages and interpretations garner the most attention and have the added perk of defensibility in the name of "vigilance."

And in the same manner in which tremendously negative predictions permit self-aggrandizing assessments of policy outcomes—such as in Neil Ferguson's claim that the lockdowns saved lives—doomy economic projections are almost always associated with unprovably optimal outcomes.[186]

An example of that is found in President Obama's assertion that without the bailouts and Fed programs administered in the wake of the 2008 financial crisis, the world might have fallen into a "permanent recession."[187] The best (and least common) unprovable counterfactuals are good guesses; the majority are deceptive.

## WHERE ECONOMISTS CAN HELP EPIDEMIOLOGISTS

Having said all of that, the paper concludes with a redemptory note, commending the efforts of epidemiology teams and warning that it would be "horrifically retrograde if this [modeling] debate ushers in a

---

186 Magness, Phillip W. 2020. "Professor Lockdown Now Claims to Have Saved 3.1 Million Lives." *American Institute for Economic Research*, June 9.

187 The idea that a "permanent recession" would have been a recession which simply lapsed into a new, permanent low level of economic activity went predictably unchallenged.

return to an era where predictions, on which huge decisions are made, are kept under lock and key (e.g. by the government—as is the case in Australia)."[188]

The mundanity of letting individuals or localities assess and act in concert with proprietary risk appetites must, on some level, be frustrating when compared with creating vast artificial populations of agents or using big data to sift through colossal data repositories. It would no doubt seem a massive waste of time to expend energy writing code and poring over results only to recommend that citizens exercise their best judgment.

Simply building and running computational models is not, of course, harmful in and of itself: it is in the leap from output to implementation where hazards emerge.[189] Here's Hayek, again, in *The Counter-Revolution of Science*:

> The universal demand for conscious control or direction of social processes is one of the most characteristic features of our generation. It expresses perhaps more clearly than any of its other cliches the peculiar spirit of the age. That anything is not consciously directed as a whole is regarded as itself a blemish, a proof of its irrationality and of the need completely to replace it by a deliberately designed mechanism... The belief that processes which are consciously directed are necessarily superior to any spontaneous process is an unfounded superstition. It

---

188 Ioannidis, Cripps, and Tanner (2020, p. 12).

189 See chapter herein entitled, "World of Warcraft's Corrupted Blood Outbreak is Not a Model for COVID-19."; See chapter herein entitled "SimCity-style Modeling Flunks the Real-World Test."

> would be truer to say [as Whitehead did] that on the contrary "civilization advances by extending the number of important operations we can perform without thinking about them."[190]

Hysterical, wildly off-the-mark forecasts about COVID-19 will ultimately cause more harm than good, and find their origins in the same set of snags which regularly trip up econometric forecasts. In the epidemiological version, instead of predicting a new Great Depression, they brought an artificial depression, a growing spate of coercive masking initiatives, school closures, and the lockdowns—which quite possibly filled the powderkeg that was ignited by the killing of George Floyd.[191] And that's what we can see, directly in front of us: the ultimate cost of surgeries foregone, rising rates of drug abuse, alcoholism, and suicides, and other knock-on effects of the ridiculous government responses to the novel coronavirus outbreak will be unfolding for a generation.[192]

What can economists teach epidemiologists? When it comes to

---

190 Hayek, F.A. 1952. *The Counter-Revolution of Science*. The Free Press: Glencoe, IL.

191 Firstpost. 2014. "How seriously should we take Roubini's doomsday predictions?" *Firstpost*, December 20; Wikipedia. 2020. "The Great Depression of 1990." *Wikipedia*, March 22.

192 Adams, Mike. 2020. "Sally Pipes: Coronavirus lockdown—How many harmed by disruption to routine medical care?" *OrthoSpineNews*, June 8; Miller, Andrew Mark. 2020. "Data shows drug overdoses soaring following virus lockdowns: Up 18% in March, 29% in April, 42% in May." *Washington Examiner*, July 2; Medical Xpress. 2020. "Lockdown prompts surge in Germans seeking help for alcoholism." *MedicalXpress*, June 4; Tucker, Jeffrey A. 2020. "Lockdown Suicide Data Reveal Predictable Tragedy." *American Institute for Economic Research*, May 22; Mohan, Megha. 2020. "Coronavirus: Domestic violence 'increases globally during lockdown.'" *BBC News*, June 12; Grasso, June. 2020. "Spike in Divorces Likely After the Lockdowns." *Bloomberg Law*, June 2; McNiff, Serena. 2020. "Lockdowns Making Things Worse for Obese Americans." *WebMD*, June 15.

forecasting, humility is key and discretion is the better part of valor. If in a position of power or influence, don't be afraid to bore politicians to death. Be aware, and remain aware, of the utter unpredictability of human action. And always, above all, remain mindful that the presence of even one human being (and more realistically, millions) introduces complexities which are difficult to predict and virtually impossible to simulate.

## DOUBTS ABOUT CONTACT TRACING

BY EDWARD P. STRINGHAM

June 17, 2020

In the movies, it all seems easy. There is a pandemic. You discover the sick person and trace where he or she has been and with whom. You notify and test those people. Find the positive cases and trace further.

In the 2011 movie *Contagion*, they find the original carrier and trace her steps back to a restaurant in China, and the chef who made her food, and the pig the chef slaughtered and then to the bat that fell into the trough.

It's science!

In real life, it's a different matter. Somehow during this pandemic, the idea of contact tracing has been held out as some sort of panacea. Your new smartphone software probably has the technology which is set to alert you if you come near someone previously seen as COVID positive or enter into some hot zone. Or if you get the virus, others will be notified of your presence—perhaps like a leper bell from the Middle Ages.

I have my doubts that most people want that on their phones but most won't know how to turn it off.[193]

Regarding these apps, Brookings writes:[194]

---

193 Potuck, Michael, 2020. "How to manage COVID-19 exposure notifications on iPhone." *9to5mac*, May 19.

194 Soltani, Ashkan, Ryan Calo, and Carl Bergstrom. 2020. "Contact-tracing apps are not a solution to the COVID-19 crisis." *Brookings,* April 27.

> The lure of automating the painstaking process of contact tracing is apparent. But to date, no one has demonstrated that it's possible to do so reliably despite numerous concurrent attempts. Apps that notify participants of disclosure could, on the margins and in the right conditions, help direct testing resources to those at higher risk. **Anything else strikes us as implausible at best, and dangerous at worst.**

Sheridan Prasso of Bloomberg offers additional insight:[195]

> Of the 47 contact-tracing apps already in use in 28 countries as of mid-May, 23% of them had no privacy policy, 53% don't disclose how long they plan to keep user data, and 60% had no publicly stated anonymity measures, *Top10VPN*'s Woodhams found. None has reached the 60% download level needed to be effective. An April white paper by the American Civil Liberties Union also said that most location-tracking methods used by apps are too inaccurate to be useful for automated tracking.
>
> A poll by Axios and Ipsos Group found 66% of respondents said they would reject an app developed by tech companies, and even more wouldn't download one from the U.S. government. "The whole concept of American democracy is about local control and civil liberties," Cliff Young, president of Ipsos U.S. Public Affairs, said in a statement with the poll results.

---

195 Prasso, Sheridan. 2020. "Everyone Has a Contact-Tracing App, and Nobody's Happy About It." *Bloomberg*, May 21.

In addition to contact tracing apps, right now governments are hiring thousands of people to work for government as detectives through widespread contact tracing. Many officials say the government must hire 300,000 (that would be one out of every thousand people in the country) to work as contact tracers.

It works as follows. Someone tests positive for COVID-19. The contact tracer then investigates where the person lives, his family and friends, and compiles a list of everyone with whom the COVID-19 patient has had contact. The contact tracer then knows everyone who has potentially been exposed and can be in touch with them.

But tracing the source and all possible people exposed to this airborne virus is easier said than done. Consider the typical New Yorker who may have in the last week been to the store twice, took delivery of packages from two UPS employees, ridden the elevator with 20 other people, and been on the subway ten times. If you touch a surface in Penn Station it may have been touched by any of the other 600,000 passengers who historically go through Penn Station, each day. Just count up all of the thousand surfaces you have touched in the past week and all the people you see.

Then what does the investigator do? The investigator makes a list, investigates for phone numbers and addresses, and taps a case worker to start making calls. "You have been in contact with someone who is COVID positive, and we would like you to come in for a test."

The contact tracer then requires that everyone potentially exposed to the virus stay home for two weeks.

Talk about a way to panic the public! Just the prospect of kicking off this incredibly invasive process might deter people from ever going to the hospital in the first place.

But let's say that you can somehow develop a map of the travels of a virus from here to there and there, and you can watch this visualization. What precisely can you do with this information? There is zero hope that you can somehow freeze all these people in place, and, even if you could, nothing about mapping and tracing causes the virus to go away.

A Yale graduate student was recently working as a contact tracer and is alerting the public about some of the downsides of how contact tracing in Connecticut is working.[196]

She found the job frustrating and didn't like poking into peoples' lives. All she was able to do was warn people and offer vague guidance. Imagine getting routine calls from government officials who "work like a detective, asking about co-workers met, errands run, shops visited, events attended" and queries like, "What did you have for breakfast, for lunch, did you go shopping, did you go to the barber shop?" And then imagine getting calls each time you were at a place that had a COVID-19 carrier. I personally like to keep my interaction with the other 4.3 million daily subway riders in New York to a minimum. What will people even be able to do with such information?

One must wonder too about the coercive aspects to this.

Q&A from Washington State offers some not very comforting assurances.[197]

---

196 Sataline, Suzanne. 2020. "Life as a Covid-19 contact tracer: sleuthing, stress, and veering off-script." *STAT*, May 18.

197 Kawash, Maher. 2020. "Debunking the myths of COVID-19 contact tracing." *KXLY*, May 14.

Q: What happens if I don't comply?

A: If health officials think you're at risk and are worried about you not complying, they'll ask you to sign a form which says you will voluntarily self-isolate. **If you still don't comply, you could face a fine or jail time**.

Q: Will I or my kids be placed in isolation centers?

A: No. The state has some isolation centers available for foster kids or people with no safe place to go. **At no point, will anyone drag you or your kids out of your home.**

Q: Why is the **National Guard involved**?

A: They are only **acting as volunteers**, not law enforcement. They will help like they are doing at the food banks in town.

Q: Will my privacy be violated?

A: No. Your information is confidential **just like it is at a doctor's office**.

Imagine being assured of the same privacy as a visit to the doctor's office, except the contact tracer tracks down and interviews everyone with whom you interacted.

Contact tracing might make sense for certain diseases. But it turns out that there is no evidence that this novel coronavirus can be contained by contact tracing.

Let us consider some of the articles on this topic:

Non-pharmaceutical public health measures for mitigating the risk and impact of epidemic and pandemic influenza.[198]

> Active contact tracing is **not recommended in general** because there is **no obvious rationale** for it in most Member States.

***Feasibility of controlling COVID-19 outbreaks by isolation of cases and contacts.***[199]

> Isolation of confirmed and suspected cases, and identification of contacts are a crucial part of these control efforts; however, **whether these efforts will achieve control of transmission of COVID-19 is unclear**… Isolation of cases and contact tracing becomes less effective if infectiousness begins before the onset of symptoms.
>
> Outbreak control was defined as no new infections between 12 and 16 weeks after the initial cases. Outbreaks that reached 5,000 cumulative cases were assumed to be too large to control within 12–16 weeks, and were categorised as uncontrolled outbreaks. Based on this definition, we reported the probability that an outbreak of a severe acute respiratory syndrome coronavirus 2-like pathogen would be controlled within 12 weeks

198 WHO. 2019. *Non-pharmaceutical public health measures for mitigating the risk and impact of epidemic and pandemic influenza.* World Health Organization.

199 Hellewell, Joel, Sam Abbott, Amy Gimma, Nikos Bosse, Christopher Jarvis, et al. 2020. "Feasibility of controlling COVID-19 outbreaks by isolation of cases and contacts." *The Lancet*, 8(4): e488-e496.

for each scenario, assuming that the basic reproduction number remained constant and no other interventions were implemented.

These outbreaks required a large number of cases to be contact traced and isolated each week, **which is of concern when assessing the feasibility of this strategy**. Subclinical infection markedly decreased the probability of controlling outbreaks within 3 months.

***Factors that make an infectious disease outbreak controllable.***[200]

We show that the success of these control measures is determined as much by the proportion of transmission occurring prior to the onset of overt clinical symptoms (or via asymptomatic infection) as the inherent transmissibility of the etiological agent (measured by the reproductive number $R_0$). From published studies, we estimate these quantities for two moderately transmissible viruses, **severe acute respiratory syndrome coronavirus and HIV**, and for two highly transmissible viruses, **smallpox and pandemic influenza**. We conclude that **severe acute respiratory syndrome and smallpox are easier to control** using these simple public health measures. Direct estimation of the proportion of asymptomatic and presymptomatic infections is achievable by contact tracing and should be a priority during an outbreak of a novel infectious agent.

---

200 Fraser, Christophe, Steven Riley, Roy M. Anderson, and Neil M. Ferguson. 2004. "Factors that make an infectious disease outbreak controllable." *PNAS,* 101(16): 6146-6151.

***Comparing nonpharmaceutical interventions for containing emerging epidemics.***[201]

The comparative effectiveness of symptom monitoring and quarantine **depends critically** on the natural history of the infectious disease, its inherent transmissibility, and the intervention feasibility in the particular healthcare setting.

***Disease contact tracing in random and clustered networks.***[202]

The efficacy of contact tracing, be it between individuals (e.g. sexually transmitted diseases or severe acute respiratory syndrome) or between groups of individuals (e.g. foot-and-mouth disease; FMD), is **difficult to evaluate without precise knowledge of the underlying contact structure**; i.e. who is connected to whom? Motivated by the 2001 FMD epidemic in the UK, we determine, using stochastic simulations and deterministic 'moment closure' models of disease transmission on networks of premises (nodes), network and disease properties that are important for contact tracing efficiency. **For random networks with a high average number of connections per node, little clustering of connections and short latency periods, contact tracing is typically ineffective**. In

---

201 Peak, Corey M., Lauren M. Childs, Yonatan H. Grad, and Caroline O. Buckee. 2017. "Comparing nonpharmaceutical interventions for containing emerging epidemics." *PNAS*, 114(15): 4023-4028.

202 Kiss, Istvan Z., Darren M. Green, and Rowland R. Kao. 2005. "Disease contact tracing in random and clustered networks." *Proceedings. Biological sciences,* 272(1570): 1407–1414.

this case, isolation of infected nodes is the dominant factor in determining disease epidemic size and duration. If the latency period is longer and the average number of connections per node small, or if the network is spatially clustered, then the contact tracing performs better and an overall reduction in the proportion of nodes that are removed during an epidemic is observed.

### *Open Letter: Contact Tracking and NHSX.*[203]

Contact tracking is unlikely to be effective in a country where not everyone has a mobile phone, and where many people live in shared accommodation—not everyone who carries the virus can or will be tracked, and cell recognition is not good enough to differentiate between people who, for instance, live in a single block of flats. **Not only does this kind of surveillance risk contravening human rights, but it is not guaranteed to work—particularly at this stage of the Coronavirus outbreak**.

In the UK, OFCOM figures show that 22% of UK adults do not have a smartphone, rising to 45% of adults over 55, and figures on device ownership for young children vary wildly.[204] Relying on this data exclusively risks reinforcing existing inequalities, especially if it could be used to establish reasonable or reliable grounds for a person to be detained.

It is not yet clear how data will be collected, or used, within

---

203 Signed by many dozens of health professionals and technologists in the UK.

204 Ofcom. 2019. "Online Nation: 2019 report." *Ofcom*, May 30.

> the legal framework. Nor what technical safeguards will be used. We are also concerned that data collected to fight Coronavirus could be stored indefinitely or for a disproportionate amount of time, or **will be used for unrelated purposes**.
>
> These are testing times, but they do not call for untested new technologies. Ethical data-driven decision-making requires good governance, transparency and willingness to course correct.

In *The Limits of Location Tracking in an Epidemic*, Jay Stanley and Jennifer Stisa Granick of the ACLU write,[205]

> At the same time, location data contains an enormously invasive and personal set of information about each of us, with the potential to reveal such things as people's social, sexual, religious, and political associations. The potential for invasions of privacy, abuse, and stigmatization is enormous.
>
> **Data on individuals' locations is not accurate enough for automated contact tracing.**
>
> We have spoken with engineers and executives at a number of the largest U.S. companies that hold location data on Americans' movements and locations, and generally they have told us that their data is not suitable for determining who was in contact with whom for purposes of COVID-19 contact tracing.
>
> The CDC warns against coming in "close contact" with a person who has tested positive for the virus, defining close

205 Stanley, Jay, and Jennifer Stisa Granick. 2020. "The Limits of Location Tracking in an Epidemic." *ACLU*, April 8.

contact as "being within approximately 6 feet (2 meters), of a person with COVID-19 for a prolonged period of time." None of the data sources discussed above are accurate enough to identify close contact with sufficient reliability. None are reliably accurate to within 6 feet. Using the wrong technology to draw conclusions about who may have become infected might lead to expensive mistakes such as two week isolation from work, friends, and family for someone—perhaps even a health care worker or first responder—who was actually not exposed. Israel's use of location data has already sparked complaints about accuracy.

**The algorithms are not likely to be reliable.**

Even if we were to imagine a set of location data that had pinpoint accuracy, there would still be problems translating that in any automated way into reliable guesses about whether two people were in danger of transmitting an infection. The Israeli system apparently acts on the basis of nothing more than an automated look at proximity. In Israel, one woman was identified as a "contact" simply because she waved at her infected boyfriend from outside his apartment building—and was issued a quarantine order based on that alone.

**The data is fragmented and may be biased.**

Complicating matters further, no single, centralized party holds the location data generated by Americans. Most location data with any level of precision is generated by an essentially corrupt ecosystem of shady, privacy-invading companies that engage in mass location tracking without individuals' meaningful awareness or consent, typically by paying the developers of smartphone apps to hide tracking capabilities inside those apps. This location data is scattered among dozens of such companies most Americans have never heard of.

**Proposed Use: Enforcement**

Another possible use of location information is in the enforcement of quarantines, shelter-in-place orders, and travel restrictions. **These uses contemplate turning people's cell phones into ersatz ankle monitors**.

Aggregate data could also be used to enforce compliance with stay-at-home orders. For example, companies could notify the authorities when cell phone data suggested that people were gathering in numbers prohibited by local public health measures, without sharing the identities of those who appear to have gathered, such as at a rogue bar that appeared in Los Angeles during a shelter-in-place regime. Such measures would have to be used with care lest multi-story apartment buildings or the like trigger alarms.

Public health experts caution, however, that a law enforcement approach to combatting disease is less effective than relying on voluntary measures and compliance. That is because an enforcement approach often sparks counterproductive resistance and evasion and tends to sour the relationship between citizens and their government at a time when trust is of paramount importance. Good public health measures leverage people's own incentives to report disease and help stop its spread.

## TECHNOCRATS SHOULD OBSERVE THE HIPPOCRATIC OATH

BY PETER C. EARLE

July 18, 2020

In some states, the lockdown reopenings are being reversed. We are seeing a new round of state versus state blame-mongering and recriminations.[206] The new benchmark for normalcy to return is January 2021. Why that date? As with many benchmarks over these months, it's completely made up.

We are supposed to believe that they know better than the rest of us, that government and not people and not medical professionals possess the essential knowledge we need.

As writer Bari Weiss commented in her July 14th *New York Times* resignation letter (albeit referring to the influence of hyper-woke Twitter intellectuals): "Truth isn't a process of collective discovery [anymore], but an orthodoxy already known to an enlightened few whose job is to inform everyone else."[207]

Local knowledge, individual risk appetites, and personal responsibility are again being supplanted by the calculations and stratagems of technocrats.

All of which reminds me of Charles McKay's *Extraordinary Delusions and the Madness of Crowds*.[208] This book focuses on financial bubbles, and a particularly interesting portion of it discusses disease

---

206 Millman, Jennifer. 2020. "22 States Now on Tri-State Quarantine List as Cuomo Ups Ante With New NY Order." *NBC New York*, July 14.

207 Weiss, Bari. 2020. Resignation Letter. *Bari Weiss*, July 14.

208 McKay, Charles. 1852. *Extraordinary Delusions and the Madness of Crowds*. London: UK.

panics as exacerbated by the forecasting experts of the early modern period. They, like their modern day descendants, thrived in an era of top-down, deferred-to expertism; not armed with massive reams of data and analytical methods at their disposal, but the similarly arcane methods of scrying and divination.

McKay sets the stage: The Great Plague of Milan, 1629 to 1631.[209] In the role that today would be occupied by the media, Hollywood, or another source of perceived wisdom, a prophecy passed down for generations held that:

> [I]n the year 1630 the devil would poison all Milan. Early one morning in April, and before the pestilence had reached its height, the passengers were surprised to see that all the doors in the principal streets of the city were marked with a curious daub, or spot, as if a sponge, filled with the purulent matter of the plague-sores, had been pressed against them. The whole population were speedily in movement to remark the strange appearance, and the greatest alarm spread rapidly. Every means was taken to discover the perpetrators, but in vain. At last the ancient prophecy was remembered, and prayers were offered up in all the churches that the machinations of the Evil One might be defeated.

Added to the fear of the disease were worries that a foreign government was at work, actively spreading the sickness.

---

209 Wikipedia. 2020. "1629–1631 Italian plague." *Wikipedia*, June 12.

> Many persons were of opinion that the emissaries of foreign powers were employed to spread infectious poison over the city; but by far the greater number were convinced that the powers of hell had conspired against them, and that the infection was spread by supernatural agencies. In the meantime the plague increased fearfully.

In a passage that reminds of early COVID-19 fears, long since dispelled:[210]

> Distrust and alarm took possession of every mind. Everything was believed to have been poisoned by the devil; the waters of the wells, the standing corn in the fields, and the fruit upon the trees. It was believed that all objects of touch were poisoned; the walls of the houses, the pavement of the streets, and the very handles of the doors. The populace were raised to a pitch of ungovernable fury.

"Snitch" policies directly reminiscent of present-day measures followed.[211]

> A strict watch was kept for the devil's emissaries, and any man who wanted to be rid of an enemy, had only to say that he had

---

210 Putterman, Samantha. 2020. "There's no evidence COVID-19 can survive on surfaces up to 17 days." *PolitiFact*, March 26.

211 Singman, Brooke. 2020. "LA Mayor Garcetti encourages residents to report violators of stay-at-home order: 'Snitches get rewards.'" *Fox News*, April 3; Bruce, Tammy. 2020. "A fascist bridge too far: Americans are asked to snitch on each other during coronavirus crisis." *Washington Times*, April 22.

> seen him besmearing a door with ointment; his fate was certain death at the hands of the mob.

Violence predictably ensued.[212]

> An old man, upwards of eighty years of age, a daily frequenter of the church of St. Antonio, was seen, on rising from his knees, to wipe with the skirt of his cloak the stool on which he was about to sit down. A cry was raised immediately that he was besmearing the seat with poison. A mob of women, by whom the church was crowded, seized hold of the feeble old man, and dragged him out by the hair of his head, with horrid oaths and imprecations. He was trailed in this manner through the mire to the house of the municipal judge, that he might be put to the rack, and forced to discover his accomplices; but he expired on the way. Many other victims were sacrificed to the popular fury.

Pity, in particular, poor Mora a "half a chemist and half a barber," accused

> …of being in league with the devil to poison Milan. His house was surrounded, and a number of chemical preparations were found. The poor man asserted, that they were intended as preservatives against infection; but some physicians, to whom they were submitted, declared they were poison. Mora was put

---

212 CBS News. 2020. "Police seen removing man from Philadelphia bus for not wearing a mask." *CBS News*, April 13; Associated News. 2020. "Coronavirus: Man killed by police after violent dispute over a face mask at Michigan store." *EuroNews*, July 15.

> to the rack, where he for a long time asserted his innocence. He confessed at last, when his courage was worn down by torture, that he was in league with the devil and foreign powers to poison the whole city; that he had anointed the doors, and infected the fountains of water. He named several persons as his accomplices, who were apprehended and put to a similar torture. They were all found guilty, and executed.

(And in an era in which statues and monuments are being pulled down or defaced, "Mora's house was [razed] to the ground, and a column erected on the spot, with an inscription to commemorate his guilt.")[213]

> While the public mind was filled with these marvellous occurrences, the plague continued to increase. The crowds that were brought together to witness the executions, spread the infection among one another. But the fury of their passions, and the extent of their credulity, kept pace with the violence of the plague; every wonderful and preposterous story was believed.

One Milanese resident described by McKay "had brooded over such tales till he became firmly convinced that the wild flights of his own fancy were realities." Telling a story about an invisible phantom chariot and demonic laboratories, a story which at any other time would have been met with derision, was suddenly (as certainly occurs today)

---

213 Schwartz, Matthew S. 2020. "Frederick Douglass Statue Torn Down On Anniversary Of Famous Speech." *NPR*, July 6; Andrea, Lawrence. 2020. "Hans Christian Heg was an abolitionist who died trying to end slavery. What to know about the man whose statue was toppled in Madison." *Milwaukee Journal Sentinel*, June 24.

infused with credibility:[214]

> [T]he minds of the people were so impressed with the idea that scores of witnesses, half crazed by disease, came forward to swear that they also had seen the diabolical stranger, and had heard his chariot, drawn by the milk-white steeds, rumbling over the streets at midnight with a sound louder than thunder. The number of persons who confessed that they were employed by the Devil to distribute poison is almost incredible.

In summary, although there was indeed a disease spreading in Milan,

> [a]n epidemic frenzy was abroad, which seemed to be as contagious as the plague. Imagination was as disordered as the body, and day after day persons came voluntarily forward to accuse themselves. They generally had the marks of disease upon them, and some died in the act of confession.

The conclusion, according to McKay? The soothsayer prophecies, "by taking away the hope of recovery—that greatest balm in any malady—increased threefold the ravages of the disease."

Looking at the lockdowns and the consequent leveling of tens and

---

214 Hinds, Julie. 2020. "Hot baths don't prevent coronavirus, and any race can get it, experts debunking rumors say." *Detroit Free Press*, March 7; McMaster, Geoff. 2020. "Why some people think COVID-19 heralds the apocalypse." *Folio*, April 24; Ogle, Connie. 2020. "These coronavirus 'cures' are faker than a bad boob job. Stop doing them now." *Miami Herald*, March 18; Cacioli, Lucas. 2020. "Bill Gates' COVID Conspiracy Grows In Italian Parliament, Allegations of Population Control by Political Anti-Vaxxer." *Blockchain News*, May 20.

perhaps hundreds of thousands of small businesses—and the myriad other costs that such a policy brings—one wonders: is there no probity?[215] It's clear that the architects of schemes will never apologize; well, not really. But will they be held accountable?[216]

Perennially, proposals are made that economists, data scientists, and other individuals with influential knowledge sets should, like medical doctors, have to take a Hippocratic Oath: an oath upholding fundamental ethics.

While the original Hippocratic Oath did not, as it does now, require physicians to "First, do no harm," the modern reach of technically-skilled elites via the media and policy should unquestionably bring that dictum.

A Technocrat's Oath would not be restrictive of the mere practice of model building, running simulations, or other present day vaticinations. Rather, it would come into force where and when the forecasts of those methods are passed to policymakers. For one thing, at least three requirements should be met; and all preferably publicly:

---

215 Sher, Leo. 2020. "The impact of the COVID-19 pandemic on suicide rates." *QJM*, June 30; Dubey, Souvik, Payel Biswas, Ritwik Ghosh, Subhankar Chatterjee, Mahua Jana Dubey, et al. 2020. "Psychosocial impact of COVID-19." *Diabetes & Metabolic Syndrome*, 14(5): 779–788; Stewart, Nikita. 2020. "Child Abuse Cases Drop 51 Percent. The Authorities Are Very Worried." *The New York Times*, June 9.

216 Tucker, Jeffrey A. 2020. "We Were Wrong: So Sorry that We Ruined Your Life." *American Institute for Economic Research*, March 28; Tucker, Jeffrey A. 2020. "At Least Some Politicians Admit Error (Sort of)." *American Institute for Economic Research*, June 19; Yang, Ethan. 2020. "Was Governor Cuomo Responsible for the Death of Thousands of Nursing Home Inhabitants?" *American Institute for Economic Research*, June 19.

1. At least three major sources of inaccuracy—whether found in deficient sources of data, questionable assumptions, or estimates of sensitivity—must be expressed clearly before and after a prediction is made;[217]
2. A discussion of statistical inference must be accompanied by a discussion of causal inference (preferably an interdisciplinary one);[218] and,
3. Any prognostication which does not prominently feature uncertainty as a growing factor over time must be summarily discarded.[219]

If professionals whose judgment can directly impact one person are bound to a strict moral code (in addition to bearing legal and reputational risk), shouldn't technocrats informing the highest levels of government face considerably more stringent standards of practice?[220]

Perhaps another of the many effects of telling two or three generations of young people that a university degree is of unquestionable value is an undue veneration of the expert class. Many of our grandparents and great-grandparents, who had a formidable assemblage of wisdom

---

217 Morgenstern, Oskar. 1963. *On the Accuracy of Economic Observations*. 2nd Ed. Princeton University Press.

218 Science Direct. 2020. "Statistical Inference." *Science Direct.*

219 Box, George. 2000. "Presentation of Uncertainty and Use of Forecasts with Explicit Uncertainty." Chapter 5 in *Forecasting Demand and Supply of Doctoral Scientists and Engineers: Report of a Workshop on Methodology* by National Research Council. Washington, DC: The National Academies Press.

220 Wright, Robert. 2019. "For Politicians, Bad Ideas are Low Risk and High Reward." *American Institute for Economic Research,* September 10.

but only a fraction of our formal schooling, were naturally doubtful in the face of boundless pessimism or optimism—especially when offered free of charge by bureaucrats from lofty heights of the Federal edifice. It was the people who lived through the Great Depression who offered such succinct quips as "You get what you pay for (and less)," and "It's always darkest before the dawn."

Whether by today's standards or a medieval one, at a certain level of influence, unqualified prognostication is either ignorant, irresponsible, or deceptive. Pithy epigrams alongside basic skepticism, knowledge of personal hygiene, and a propensity to self-isolate in the face of illness have superintended the human relationship with microorganisms more than massive agent-based models ever will.

## WHY DID THEY CLOSE THE SCHOOLS?

### BY JEFFREY TUCKER

June 8, 2020

On March 12, 2020, a banshee-like cry went out to an email list of public health professionals and government officials who were then in a state of mental meltdown. Pull the trigger now, screamed the memo. Close the schools.

As with any email chain, there were a few dominant voices who post more than others and with more passion, while others shrink back in fear of being shamed. Such was the case here: one disciple of computer modeling, Dr. Carter Mecher of the Veterans Administration, was convinced that the coronavirus was another Spanish Flu.

Why? He didn't explain. Mostly he wanted to try out his closure/lockdown/social-distance model on which he had been working for 14 years since he first became a convert to agent-based modeling techniques. Coronavirus of 2020 was as good an excuse as any.

Mecher emerged as the leader of the list, sending hundreds of messages of increasing alarm. Others had already joined in the alarm party. *The New York Times*'s Daniel McNeil had two weeks earlier publicly predicted as many as 8.25 million Americans would die, meaning 5 of your friends.[221] He knew this because this virus "reminded" him of the Spanish Flu too.

Mecher, a longtime pusher of the cooties theory of viruses (in which running and hiding is always the answer), called for an immediate nationwide school closing, even though it was already apparent that

221 Tucker, Jeffrey A. 2020. "Why Does the New York Times Deny the Obvious?" *American Institute for Economic Research*, June 5.

COVID-19 represented almost zero threat to school kids.

Pull the trigger now, he demanded. Do it all at once, now, attaching his long document filled with startling pictures of mass death and how school closures would stop that. It's no big deal, he promised. Kids love being home. It will bring families together (so long as they stay six feet apart).

Within days it happened. Then the dominos began to fall. If kids are home, parents have to be also. Offices and stores should close too. If they are older, they will congregate in malls and parks, so they must close too. So too amusement parks, bowling alleys, aquariums, museums, and anything but the most essential businesses.

In the blink of an eye, a nation locked down. Let us remember that it began domestically (Trump had already and stupidly banned international travel) with the schools, schools on which kids depend for education and social connection and parents pay for in taxes and tuition. States, without warning and with only evidence of crazed and fearful frenzy, shut their doors, thus sending tens of millions home and disrupting the lives of every American household.

On May 1, 2020, the prestige journal *The Lancet* said the following:[222]

> Currently, the evidence to support national closure of schools to combat COVID-19 is very weak and data from influenza outbreaks suggest that school closures could have relatively small effects on a virus with COVID-19's high transmissibility

---

222 Viner, Russell M., Simon J. Russell, Helen Croker, Jessica Packer, Joseph Ward, et al. 2020. "School closure and management practices during coronavirus outbreaks including COVID-19: a rapid systematic review." *The Lancet* 4(5): 397-404.

> and apparent low clinical effect on school children. At the same time, these data also show that school closures can have profound economic and social consequences.

Whoops. So far as I know, Carter Mecher has had nothing to say these days.

Within Maryland, a wonderful group of activists put out a document explaining why all of this is a terrible idea. The manifesto of Reopen-Maryland group is an impressive document.[223]

* * *

Schools across the country have closed since the novel coronavirus, which causes the disease known as COVID-19, emerged in the U.S. But what does the data really say about school closure and reopening related to COVID-19?

## DO EXPERTS BELIEVE SCHOOLS SHOULD REMAIN CLOSED?

A recent analysis in the Lancet concluded the evidence for national school closure due to COVID-19 was "very weak" and would have "profound economic and social consequences" while providing a relatively minor (2-4%) reduction in overall death rates.[224] The Centers for Disease Control and Prevention (CDC) recently released a decision tree

---

223 2020. "Reopen Maryland." *Reopen-Maryland.com*

224 Viner, Russell M., Simon J. Russell, Helen Croker, Jessica Packer, Joseph Ward, Claire Stansfield, Oliver Mytton, Chris Bonell & Robert Booy. 2020. "School closure and management practices during coronavirus outbreaks including COVID-19: a rapid systematic review." *The Lancet*, 4(5).

suggesting schools should reopen as long as local ordinances allowed it, staff had capacity to screen for COVID-19 symptoms and schools had adequate personal protective equipment for staff who needed it.[225] A recent discussion among education heads in the European Union concluded that school reopening there had not led to spikes in cases.[226]

## IS IT SAFE TO REOPEN SCHOOLS?

The WHO's chief scientist says children seem "less capable" of spreading coronavirus and are at "very low risk" of illness.[227] The same scientist reports that no major outbreaks have resulted from school reopening. Multiple studies have found that, while it remains theoretically possible for children to transmit the virus to adults, it occurs far less frequently than originally feared. Studies of transmission within families found children "unlikely" to have passed the virus to adults in their own households.[228]

## EVEN IF COMMUNITY SPREAD OCCURRED IN SCHOOLS, HOW DEADLY IS COVID-19?

COVID-19 is far less deadly than originally predicted, with the risk of death, for adults, roughly equivalent to the risk of death from driving

---

225 Centers for Disease Control and Prevention (CDC). 2020. "Schools during the COVID-19 pandemic."

226 Boffey, Daniel, & Kim Willsher. 2020. "Schools reopening has not triggered rise in Covid-19 cases, EU ministers told." *The Guardian*, May 18.

227 British Broadcasting Corporation. 2020. "Children 'seem less capable of spreading virus.'" *BBC*, May 17.

228 Boast, Alison, Alistair Munro, & Henry Goldstein. 2020. "An evidence summary of Paediatric COVID-19 literature. Don't Forget the Bubbles." At p. 5.

a car.[229] The risk to children is even lower; children accounted for fewer than 2% of total COVID-19 cases in a large CDC study, and of those children who did contract the virus, a maximum of 2% required hospitalization.[230] In one study, most admissions to pediatric intensive care units involved children with "significant preexisting comorbidities."[231] While some cases of a rare inflammatory complication have been reported, cases remain uncommon and schools are not closed for similar post-infectious inflammatory syndromes such as Kawasaki disease.[232] Pediatric deaths from COVID-19 are "extremely rare."[233] In fact, one study cautioned that far from reducing mortality, closing schools due to COVID-19 might actually increase mortality, increasing absenteeism among the healthcare workforce and thereby placing strain on the healthcare system.[234]

---

229 Ioannidis, John P.A., Catherine Axfors, & Despina G. Contopoulos-Ioannidis. 2020. "Population-level COVID-19 mortality risk for non-elderly individuals overall and for non-elderly individuals without underlying diseases in pandemic epicenters." *Environmental Research*, 188.

230 Centers for Disease Control and Prevention COVID-19 Response Team. 2020. "Coronavirus disease 2019 in children—United States, February 12–April 2, 2020." *Morbidity and Mortality Weekly Report*, 69: 422–426.

231 Shekerdemian, Lara S., Nabihah R. Mahmood, Katie K. Wolfe, K., Beckie J. Riggs, Catherine E. Ross et al. 2020. "Characteristics and outcomes of children with coronavirus disease 2019 (COVID-19) infection admitted to US and Canadian pediatric intensive care units." *JAMA Pediatrics*. Published online May 11.

232 European Centre for Disease Prevention and Control. 2020. "Rapid risk assessment: Paediatric inflammatory multisystem syndrome and SARS-CoV-2 infection in children." May 15.

233 Boast, Munro & Goldstein (2020, p.4).

234 Bayhem, Jude, & Eli P. Fenichel. 2020. "Impact of school closures for COVID-19 on the US health-care workforce and net mortality: a modelling study." *The Lancet*, April 3.

## HAVE OTHER COUNTRIES SAFELY REOPENED SCHOOLS?

Some countries such as Taiwan never closed schools, and many others, including 22 European countries, have reopened without significant spikes in children's infections.[235]

## HOW EFFECTIVE IS "SOCIALLY DISTANCED" LEARNING?

Evidence suggests that remote learning can be less effective than face-to-face learning for many schoolchildren, including those with special education needs, as intensive therapies often cannot be delivered remotely.[236] In fact, socially distanced learning is likely to cause a "historic academic regression" that will particularly disadvantage these students, as well as students from backgrounds of poverty and students learning English.[237] In addition, concerns abound about the developmental appropriateness of socially distanced learning for young children in particular.[238] Recent guidelines from the CDC for socially distanced school resumption, for example, present recommendations that are challenging to implement in developmentally and socially

---

235 Boffey & Willsher (2020); McFall-Johnsen, Morgan. 2020. "School closures may not help prevent the spread of the coronavirus, and some experts say they may do more harm than good." *Business Insider*, May 13.

236 Robles, Yesenia. 2020. "Amid coronavirus fears, the CDC told schools to plan for remote learning. That's harder than it sounds." *Chalkbeat.org,* March 3; Leone, Hannah, & Karen Ann Cullotta. 2020. Coronavirus school shutdown has been particularly tough on kids with special needs: 'It's not just a disruption. We're going to see kids who actually go backward.' *Chicago Tribune*, April 27.

237 Richards, Erin. 2020. "'Historic academic regression:' Why homeschooling is so hard amid school closures." *USA Today*, April 13.

238 Silverman, Amy. 2020. "Play, child development, and relationships: A preschool teacher in China shares her virtual teaching experience." *Teaching Young Children*, 13(4).

appropriate ways.[239] These include steps such as universal playground closure, seating that does not allow for collaboration or discussion, and restriction of movement in the classroom.

## HOW DO SCHOOL CLOSURES IMPACT ACADEMIC GROWTH?

Spring 2020 closures are projected to place students 30-50% behind where they would otherwise have been, with more significant loss in math.[240] Some students will have lost almost a full year of growth from spring alone, with any fall closures increasing this gap.[241] Numerous experts agree school closure poses significant academic risks.[242] In addition, options for partial or staggered school reopenings may impact students' academic progress and well-being in yet-unquantified ways.

## HOW DO SCHOOL CLOSURES IMPACT STUDENTS WHO NEED ADDITIONAL SUPPORT?

School closure and related interruptions to learning hit academically vulnerable students hardest.[243] Those with disabilities cannot access needed services and often receive developmentally inappropriate and ineffective online learning in place of the intensive personal therapies

---

239 Centers for Disease Control and Prevention (CDC). 2020. "CDC activities and initiatives supporting the COVID-19 response and the president's plan for opening America up again." *CDC*, May.

240 Kuhfeld, Megan, James Soland, Beth Tarasawa, Angela Johnson, Erik Ruzek & Jing Liu. 2020. "Projecting the potential impacts of COVID-19 school closures on academic achievement." *Brown University, Annenberg Institute* Ed-WorkingPaper No. 20-226.

241 Christakis, Dimitri A. 2020. "School reopening—the pandemic issue that is not getting its due." *JAMA Pediatrics*, May 13.

242 Ibid.

243 Kuhfeld et al. (2020).

they need.[244] Additionally, a recent Lancet article predicted COVID-19 related school closures are likely to "exacerbate food insecurity" and "widen the learning gap" for students from backgrounds of poverty.[245]

## HOW DO SCHOOL CLOSURES IMPACT STUDENTS' SAFETY?

Abuse cases, including some reported fatalities, have been on the rise since school closure and lockdown orders. Teachers are often the first to report suspected child abuse, and states have reported a drop in these referrals since COVID-19 related school closures.[246] In fact, researchers estimated that over 200,000 claims of child abuse across the nation may have gone unreported in March and April 2020 due to school closures.[247] While not all claims of abuse are substantiated or suggest imminent harm, it is certain that children in dangerous or vulnerable home situations are left without needed support when schools are closed. Additionally, reports indicate that the COVID-19 shutdowns have increased the risk of substance abuse as well as mental health issues, with adolescents being particularly vulnerable to addiction.[248]

---

244 Adely, Hannan. 2020. "'No one to help me:' Special education families struggle with coronavirus school closures." *USA Today,* April 23.

245 Van Lancker, W., & Parolin, Z. 2020. COVID-19, school closures, and child poverty: a social crisis in the making. *The Lancet*. Public health, 5(5), e243–e244. At p.1)

246 Richardson, Ryann. 2020. "School closures affect rates of reported child abuse." *Standard-Examiner*, May 15.

247 Barron, Jason E., Ezra G. Goldstein, & Cullen T. Wallace. 2020. "Suffering in silence: How COVID-19 school closures inhibit the reporting of child maltreatment." *Social Science Research Network*, May 14.

248 Panchal, Nirmita, Rabah Kamal, Kendal Orgera, Cynthia Cox, Rachel Garfield, et al. 2020. "The implications of COVID-19 for mental health and substance use." *KFF*, April 21.

## HOW DO SCHOOL CLOSURES IMPACT STUDENTS' MENTAL HEALTH?

There is widespread agreement that school closure is harmful to children's mental health, with parents reporting increased depression, stress, anxiety and suicidal ideation.[249] A recent study of child mental health during China's lockdown found increased symptoms of anxiety and depression, for example.[250] Another study found 83% of young people with mental health needs reported their conditions worsening during the pandemic.[251]

## HOW DO SCHOOL CLOSURES IMPACT THE ECONOMY?

The economic impact of school closure and interruptions to learning are substantial and harmful. One analysis, for example, found extended school closure for pandemic illness can reduce Gross Domestic Product (GDP) by over $100 billion.[252] School closure wastes school system resources and causes workforce disruptions, affecting 16-30% of the workforce, with higher impact in healthcare.[253] Concerns are now being

---

249 Kamenetz, Anya. 2020. "With school buildings closed, children's mental health is suffering." *NPR*, May 14.

250 Xie, Xinyan, Qi Xue, & Yu Zhou. 2020. "Mental health status among children in home confinement during the coronavirus disease 2019 outbreak in Hubei Province, China." *JAMA Pediatrics,* April 24.

251 Lee, Joyce. 2020. "Mental health effects of school closures during COVID-19." *The Lancet*, April 14.

252 Lempel, Howard, Ross A. Hammond, & Joshua M. Epstein. 2009. "Costs of school closure." *Brookings Institute*, September 30.

253 Lempel, Howard, Joshua M. Epstein, & Ross A. Hammond Epstein. 2009. "Economic cost and health care workforce effects of school closures in the U.S." *PLoS currents*, 1, RRN1051; Sadique, M. Z., Adams, E. J., & Edmunds, W. J. (2008). Estimating the costs of school closure for mitigating an influenza pandemic. *BMC public health*, 8, 135.

raised about heightened risks for school dropout among adolescents whose education has been interrupted.[254] Those who drop out of high school are far less likely to find employment and far more likely to become involved with the correctional system.[255]

## WHAT KIND OF MEASURES SHOULD WE TAKE TO REOPEN SCHOOLS?

Schools and districts will need to identify ways to protect vulnerable teachers and staff through flexible scheduling and staffing, and schools and districts will likewise need to make provisions for medically vulnerable students to continue to learn with appropriate health protections or remote accommodations. Within schools, some common-sense measures have been proposed, such as frequent handwashing, screening students and staff for illness, and meticulous cleaning.[256] Such steps are minimally disruptive to adopt. However, recent guidance from the CDC presents recommendations whose scope is far more than minimally disruptive, such as closing playgrounds, requiring masks for children over 2, cancelling extracurricular activities, and restricting movement

---

254 Torres, Stacy. 2020. "After coronavirus, expect high school dropout wave. 9/11 was the trigger for my sisters." *USA Today*, 30 April.

255 Department of Labor. 2019. "44.6 percent of high school dropouts and 72.3 percent of college graduates employed in August 2019." *U.S. Bureau of Labor Statistics*, September 11; Berger-Gross, Andrew. 2020. "From school to prison: The criminal justice outcomes of youth with disabilities in North Carolina." *North Carolina Department of Commerce*, January 27.

256 Mineo, Liz. 2020. "How to reduce the spread of coronavirus." *The Harvard Gazette*, March 5; Centers for Disease Control and Prevention (CDC). 2020. "Considerations for Schools." *CDC*, May 19.

in the classroom.[257] Such practices have uncertain basis in the literature while being likely to have significant impact on students' academic, socioemotional and neurological development. Recent research found that teachers expressed significant concerns about feasibility of practices such as canceling recess, restricting student movement in the classroom, and staggering days.[258] The CDC's recommendation to restrict attendance to students from certain localities presents significant legal challenges with respect to charter school and magnet program students, those attending out-of-area vocational or English language programs, and (in particular) students with special education needs who require specialized instruction in highly supported programs outside their neighborhood schools.[259] In general, recommendations for social distancing within schools must be evaluated in light of their developmental appropriateness and impact on academic and socio-emotional growth, especially given the minimal risk that COVID-19 appears to pose to children.

## CONCLUSION

In many respects, school-aged children have borne the brunt of our social response to the coronavirus pandemic. While not often at direct

---

257 Centers for Disease Control and Prevention (2020, "CDC activities and initiatives supporting the COVID-19 response and the president's plan for opening America up again").

258 Uscher-Pines, Lori, Heather L. Schwartz, Faruque Ahmed, Yenlik Zheteyeva, Jennifer Tamargo Leschitz et al. 2020. "Feasibility of Social Distancing Practices in US Schools to Reduce Influenza Transmission During a Pandemic." *Journal of Public Health Management and Practice.*

259 Centers for Disease Control and Prevention (2020, "CDC activities and initiatives…").

risk of harm from the virus itself, students have seen their educational trajectories significantly disrupted, with undeniable academic, physical, social and mental health impact. Alternatives being proposed for fall, such as remote or hybrid learning, hold little promise to rectify these disastrous impacts or provide any sense of stability to America's schoolchildren. If anything, options such as hybrid instruction, "socially distanced" classes with desks six feet apart, and school days with minimal social contact all promise to further disrupt students' learning and undermine the sense of stability that is critical to healthy child and adolescent development. In the face of increasingly clear research on the impact of school closure, we must seriously consider the question of competing harms. Closures offer uncertain and relatively minor benefits in overall pandemic control, but their harms to children and society at large are known and significant. As we emerge from this period of national crisis, reopening schools can prove an effective way to help repair our strained social fabric. School helps to guarantee educational access and equal opportunity. School helps to facilitate students' cognitive and academic development, to support social and emotional connection, and to re-establish valuable routines for children and adults alike. For the well-being of our nation's children and our society at large, it is critical that decision-makers immediately prioritize children's timely return to school so that all of our nation's children can access the high-quality, developmentally appropriate educational experience that they undeniably deserve.

The Reopen Schools Project at Reopen Maryland has the goal of furthering equitable, effective and data-based policies and programming for students within Maryland and across the country in the wake of coronavirus-related school closures. Long-term closures have disrupted educational access and well-being for millions of children and adolescents, creating potential for significant and lasting social, economic and educational damage. The Reopen Schools Project advocates for evidence-based decision-making that incorporates an accurate understanding of all relevant variables, including health and epidemiological considerations, mental health, social and physical development, educational equity, academic growth, and social stability.

## FAUCI IS WRONG: NEW YORK DID NOT DO IT "CORRECTLY"

BY PETER C. EARLE AND FIONA HARRIGAN

July 23, 2020

After a months-long struggle to contain COVID-19, New York Governor Andrew Cuomo seems confident that he has steered the state to safety at long last. He has hardly shied away from expressing pride over his pandemic policies, spurring headlines that derided his "gaslighting" and his "cringeworthy victory lap."[260]

And Cuomo landed squarely in the good graces of White House health advisor Dr. Anthony Fauci, who, on July 18, lauded New York State's handling of the crisis.

Fauci declared, "They did it correctly."[261]

This interpretation was curious, given that the state's pandemic prevention efforts have been marred by grave errors.[262]

Those errors became the subject of deep scrutiny in a recent academic article entitled, "A Case Study in Model Failure? COVID-19 Daily

---

260 Harsanyi, David. 2020. "Don't fall for Cuomo's gaslighting on coronavirus." *The Star Democrat*, July 21; Greenman, Josh. 2020. "Cuomo's cringeworthy COVID victory lap." New York Daily News, July 13.

261 Dzhanova, Yelena. 2020. "Fauci holds up New York as model for fighting coronavirus — 'They did it correctly.'" *CNBC*, July 30.

262 Yang, Ethan. 2020. "Was Governor Cuomo Responsible for the Death of Thousands of Nursing Home Inhabitants?" *American Institute for Economic Research*, June 19; see article herein entitled "The Real Pandemic Was a Nursing Home Problem."

Deaths and ICU Bed Utilisation Predictions for New York State."[263]

Written by a team of mathematicians, biostatisticians, and data scientists from Stanford University, the University of Texas at El Paso, Northwestern University, and the University of Sydney, the paper takes direct aim at the decision support tools—models—that were influential in shaping New York State's policy response to the disease spread.

The four models reviewed are those produced by the Institute for Health Metrics and Evaluation (IHME), Youyang Gu, the University of Texas at Austin, and the Los Alamos National Laboratory. Though they were widely cited and enthusiastically implemented, these models fell short:

> Forecasting models have been influential in shaping decision-making in the COVID-19 pandemic. However, there is concern that their predictions may have been misleading. Here we dissect the predictions made by four models for the daily COVID-19 death counts between March 24 and June 5 in New York State, as well as the predictions of ICU bed utilisation made by the influential IHME [Institute of Health Metrics and Evaluations] model. We evaluated the accuracy of the point estimates and the accuracy of the uncertainty estimates of the model predictions … For accuracy of prediction, all models fared very poorly. Only 10.2% of the predictions fell within 10% of their training ground truth, irrespective of distance into the future … For ICU bed utilisation, the IHME model was

263 Chin, Vincent, Noelle I. Samia, Roman Marchant, Ori Rosen, John P.A. Ioannidis, Martin A. Tanner, and Sally Cripps. 2020. "A Case Study in Model Failure? COVID-19 Daily Deaths and ICU Bed Utilisation Predictions in New York State." *arXiv.*

> highly inaccurate; the point estimates only started to match ground truth after the pandemic wave had started to wane.

As COVID-19 first began to spread, ICU bed predictions were indeed dire. In March, Governor Cuomo declared that New York would require between 18,600 and 37,200 ICU beds to treat the impending wave of COVID-19 cases.[264] Compare that to New York's reality: 3,000 ICU beds available as of Cuomo's assessment. If these horrific prophecies came true, the state's medical system would have been entirely overwhelmed. It was these concerns, driven by model predictions, that informed the strategy that came to be known as "flattening the curve:" attempting to preserve medical resources by blunting the rush of all but the most dire COVID-19 cases to hospitals and healthcare facilities.

How did the models backing the curve-flattening perform?

> The accuracy of point estimates—which is to say, the actual daily death count predictions generated by each model—is evaluated using two metrics: the mean absolute percentage error and the maximum allowable percentage error. The former, in a straightforward way, calculates the percentage difference between a given model's prediction for a specific day and the actual result on that day. The latter takes the maximum of the absolute percentage errors for each forecast and each model.

The authors of the paper find that "while some models may perform better or worse over subsets of the time frame of interest, no one model

264 Shapiro, Ariel. 2020. "Cuomo Says New York Needs As Many As 37,000 ICU Beds; Unfortunately, It Has Only 3,000." *Forbes*, Mar 17.

clearly dominates throughout [the time period] with respect to either of the metrics." Across them, only 10.2% of the daily death predictions fall within 10% of the actual outcomes.

Of the paper's two major findings, one is nontrivial but unsurprising: the methods of data collection and the verification of data quality exercise great influence over models. Poor data makes good models bad, and bad models worse. A related issue arises:

> [e]arly on, Dr. Anthony Fauci, NIAID Director, stated that: "As I've told you on the show, models are really only as good as the assumptions that you put into the model. But when you start to see real data, you can modify that model..." An open question raised ... is how can one expect quality predictions, if the data are faulty? ... Clearly, if the data are suspect, projections may also be sub-optimal.

The second conclusion, of considerably more gravity, bears repeating:

> Models need to be subjected to real-time performance tests, before their results are provided to policy makers and public health officials. In this paper, we provide examples of such tests, but irrespective of which tests are adopted, they need to be specified in advance, as one would do in a well-run clinical trial.

Only the Los Alamos National Laboratory model "was found to approach the 95% nominal coverage," but it was not available when Cuomo was forging his March policy decisions. Furthermore, a model that gradually becomes more accurate is functionally irrelevant, given that it is in the early stages of a pandemic that sound and timely decisions are paramount.

Such dire ICU bed utilization predictions never came to pass,[265] at least not to the degree that was so widely feared, but the sense of urgency surrounding them compelled New York State leadership to prepare accordingly. The models were run, their purveyors advised, and policymakers listened.

Thousands of recovering coronavirus patients were sent to nursing homes, landing in settings that even Cuomo has called "the optimum feeding ground for this virus."[266] Moving elderly COVID-19 patients back into nursing homes—which produced a contagion effect that has been likened to "fire through dry grass"—was done in the name of flattening the curve, keeping hospital beds and other resources from being overwhelmed as the initial spread proceeded.[267] But devastation followed. As of July 15, 42 percent of all U.S. deaths were linked to nursing homes, amounting to more than 57,000 lives lost—over 6,000 of them in New York.[268]

Needless to say, there will be no recognition of the role that awful models played in the formulation of practices that extinguished so many innocent lives. Real-time evaluation of prediction models would

---

265 Feuer, Alan, and Jesse McKinley. 2020. "Virus Deaths Mount, but N.Y. Avoids Predicted Surge at Hospitals So Far." *The New York Times*, April 10.

266 Condon, Bernard, Jennifer Peltz, and Jim Mustian. 2020. "AP count: Over 4,500 virus patients sent to NY nursing homes." *AP News*, May 22.

267 Sapien, Joaquin, and Joe Sexton. 2020. "'Fire Through Dry Grass': Andrew Cuomo Saw COVID-19's Threat to Nursing Homes. Then He Risked Adding to It." *ProPublica*, June 16.

268 NYT. 2020. "More Than 40% of U.S. Coronavirus Deaths Are Linked to Nursing Homes." *The New York Times*, July 15.

allow policymakers and medical experts to arrive at better prevention methods if their established plan of attack was proven inaccurate—or at the very least, they could tailor the rigidity of policy responses to the evinced exactness of outcomes. But such an approach was clearly absent in New York State. In terms of predictions of hospital resources being utilized, the degree of error between forecasts and reality was so great that it could have counterbalanced the fervor with which nursing home residents were sent back to those facilities to preserve hospital beds.

Not long after that decision, adding deep insult to unfathomable injury,

> [i]n the chaotic days of late March, as it became clear that New York was facing a catastrophic outbreak of the coronavirus, aides to Gov. Andrew M. Cuomo quietly inserted a provision on Page 347 of New York's final, voluminous budget bill. Many lawmakers were unaware of the language when they approved the budget a few days later. But it provided unusual legal protections for an influential industry that has been devastated by the crisis: nursing home operators.[269]

In light of these findings, it's difficult to determine which is more of an affront to the families of the thousands upon thousands of victims of New York State's handling of COVID-19. Is it the shameless self-aggrandizing and celebration by Cuomo, whose policies led to the devastation of the elderly in long-term care facilities? Is it Dr. Anthony Fauci's commendation of those policies? Or is it the legal protection of the entities that abetted such widespread demise?

---

269 2020. "In March, Cuomo Quietly Slipped In Liability Protections To Shield Hard-Hit Nursing Homes From Lawsuits." *Kaiser Health News*, May 14.

Ultimately, there is plenty of blame to go around. But one thing is certain: the deep human costs of this virus and its corresponding policies have been exacerbated by blind hubris and unfounded pride—which, to no small extent, saw their expression in the conceit of rule by models. Though it might be too little too late, diligent reflection and readjustment in future pandemic combat efforts will be the only way to honor those who were lost so unnecessarily.[270]

270 See article herein entitled "What Economists Can Teach Epidemiologists."

## WHO IS MAKING DECISIONS ABOUT OUR LIVES

BY DONALD J. BOUDREAUX

July 13, 2020

Opinions vary enormously about the merits of government-imposed lockdowns in response to the coronavirus. Some data get flung here, other data are paraded there, all amidst fiery discussions of the reality and relative importance of concepts that most of us had never heard of until just a few months ago—concepts such as herd immunity, comorbidity, T-cells, and the flattening of curves. Conclusions differing as starkly from each other as night differs from day are drawn, with ardent champions of each conclusion insisting that his or her stance is the one—the *only* one—justified by "science."

### SCIENCE CANNOT TELL US HOW TO MAKE TRADE-OFFS

By now, it's become trite (but still true!) in the pages of sensible publications to note that the question of whether or not government should lock down the economy—and, if so, to what extent—is not one that can be answered by science. Science, of course, supplies information that is highly useful for choosing a course of action. How contagious is the coronavirus? How lethal *is* COVID-19? Do the health effects of this disease strike different age groups differently? What's the likelihood of a vaccine becoming available within the next year? Within the next two years?

Scientific questions all. And, of course, the ones listed here are only a small sample of the complete set of relevant questions. But ask as many such questions as are appropriate, and answer each as thoroughly and as accurately as would Einstein, and you'll find no answer to the Big Question: What should government do in response to the coronavirus?

To competently answer this Big Question requires knowledge that science cannot deliver. One of the most important (although not the only) species of knowledge that is scientifically undeliverable is knowledge of the preferences and risk tolerances of hundreds of millions of individuals. Preferences, including that for risk, are subjective and, hence, cannot even in principle be measured objectively. And these preferences change over time as people learn and gain new experiences.

In addition, preferences differ from person to person. The value that Betsy attaches to the freedom to reopen her retail store differs from the value that Barry puts on being able to return to his job on the factory floor. But if Betsy and Barry are under the jurisdiction of the same government, each must suffer or enjoy, as the case might be, whatever policy that government follows. To recognize that reducing the risk of exposure to coronavirus involves trade-offs, and to recognize also that the appropriate trade-off for Betsy almost certainly differs from that for Barry, is to recognize the absurdity of believing that determining the best government policy is a matter of science.

## THE TRACK RECORD IS NOT ENCOURAGING

Nevertheless, government must do something regarding COVID and the economy, even if the 'something' done is nothing. I confess to *strongly* leaning in the direction of having government do nothing. And my reason for this strong leaning is summarized by the two words "These People"—as in "What good reason have we to believe that these people in high government positions will make sensible decisions?"

These People are politically driven. Even *if* (contrary to fact) there were a scientifically determinable single best course of government action in this crisis, what reason have These People given us to believe that they are capable of finding that course and of understanding it? And even *if* These People could find and understand this scientifically 'best' course of action, what reason have we to believe that they possess the political fortitude to implement and stick to it?

More fundamentally, These People have an atrocious track record when it comes to the economy. These People routinely display appalling ignorance of the most basic facts of economic reality.

These People regularly act as if the world is filled with free lunches and as if reality is optional.

When they raise minimum wages, These People deny that low-skilled workers will suffer any negative consequences. When they raise tariffs, These People proclaim that the resulting greater scarcities at home will bring about greater abundance. When they defend rent control, These People, applauding themselves for helping poor families, remain oblivious to the resulting reduced availability and worsening quality of rental housing.

These People concoct in their political petri dishes the economic cancer of occupational licensing and then unleash it on society. In doing so, These People see only the increased incomes of the monopolists whose competitors are killed off. These People are blind to the harm suffered both by consumers and by those producers denied the opportunity to offer their services to the public.

These People defend the government-school monster-monopoly. They pump ever-more taxpayer money into this monster's maw and insist that the monster's continuing failures justify not ridding it of its monopoly status but, instead, stuffing it with ever-more taxpayer money.

These People seem not to understand the first thing about incentives.

These People either actively support or do nothing to oppose the calamitous "war on drugs." This fact shouldn't surprise, I guess: after all, These People profit from the banana republic practice of civil asset forfeiture—a practice These People declare to be an important "tool" in fighting the "war on drugs."

Very many of These People believe that adults are children who, absent the kindly intervention of These People, will guzzle too many sugary drinks, ingest too many trans fats, and vape excessively.

These People insist that the typical American is too irresponsible to save for his or her own retirement. Yet many of These People cannot arrange for the government in which they serve to live within its own means. These People spend borrowed money like mad today and, without shame—or, maybe worse, without realizing it—pass the bill on to future generations. These People clearly haven't the backbone to deny the most frivolous and costly goodies to their constituents. These People, after all, won't be in office when the bills come due—so what do These People care about what happens in the future?

These People incessantly display utter ignorance of—or contempt for—basic economic realities. These People have done so for generations. Much of what These People say about economic matters is the economic equivalent of voodoo, and even more of what they do on the economic front is destructive. And These People are none too careful with facts: They frequently stoke fears, on the flimsiest of evidence, of looming calamities whenever doing so seems to justify their seizing more power.

What reason is there to trust that These People—whose incentives are never to look past the next election and to ignore consequences that are difficult to see if these consequences are spread over large numbers of individuals—are making a prudently considered trade-off between the lockdown's costs and its benefits?

Why in the world should we trust with the power to lock down an economy These People?

## HOW A FREE SOCIETY DEALS WITH PANDEMICS, ACCORDING TO LEGENDARY EPIDEMIOLOGIST AND SMALLPOX ERADICATOR DONALD HENDERSON

BY EDWARD P. STRINGHAM

May 21, 2020

Economists have been writing for hundreds of years on the role of government in solving economic and social problems. A theme has emerged throughout: policy officials are quite often ill-informed or have bad incentives compared with what individuals, markets, institutions, and society can achieve on their own. Economists have documented how government intervention leads to various unintended economic consequences and even human rights abuses.

We prefer private governance to public governance. We have applied this logic against socialism, fascism, war, macroeconomic planning, public goods, monetary policy, countercyclical fiscal policy, environmental regulation, and a hundred other issues. We've made a solid case for pure freedom.

And yet here we are living in times when the state is controlling our movements, shuttering businesses, defining who and what is essential, dangerously disrupting supply chains, forcibly closing schools and churches, and restricting travel. A shelter-in-place order is something of a liberal nightmare, the worst-possible use of coercive power against individual rights, and the results have been catastrophic.

It's my view that we have been ill-prepared to deal with this onslaught. We have a very thin record of writings that make the case that freedom, market forces, and private governance are better than government quarantines and closures in dealing with pandemics. So where do we turn for better arguments and a better case?

Part of the problem is that as economists, historians, and political philosophers people are telling us to stay in our lane and not comment on medical matters. In general that is good advice. But there is a problem. The computer scientists and theoretical physicists who dreamed up this lock down haven't really had serious medical training either and they sure haven't stayed in their lane. They certainly have cared very little for the economic implications of their plans.

Where do we turn for competent commentary on the medical aspects of quarantine and lockdowns? Where is our credentialled and experienced expert who can provide weighty evidence that this is the wrong course?

Let me introduce you to Donald A. Henderson (1928-2016). He was the twentieth-century's most acclaimed disease eradicator. In particular, he is credited with ridding the world of smallpox. He was born in Lakewood, Ohio, son of a nurse and an engineer. He went to Oberlin College for undergraduate and graduated in medicine from the University of Rochester. He trained two more years at the Epidemic Intelligence Service of the Communicable Disease Center, and moved to Geneva to head the World Health Organization's division focussed on smallpox.

I encourage you to read his entire biography posted at Johns Hopkins, where he headed a brilliant epidemiological team.[271]

In 2006, at the order of the Bush administration, some computer science programmers with a small group of public health officials began to resurrect a premodern idea of quarantines, closures, and measured lockdowns. This way of thinking is not just premodern; it turned the logic of modern medicine on its head. It was based on a theory that we should just run away from viruses, whereas Dr. Henderson's whole

---

271 JHSPC. N.d. "Donald Ainslie Henderson MD, MPH '60." *Johns Hopkins Bloomberg School of Public Health.*

life had been devoted to implementing the great discovery of modern virus theory that we need not flee but rather build immunity through science, either natural immunities or via vaccines.

At the age of 78, Dr. Henderson swung into action and composed a masterful response to the new fashion for quarantines and lockdowns. The result was "Disease Mitigation Measures in the Control of Pandemic Influenza."[272] Henderson, though listed last, was the primary author along with co-authors Thomas V. Inglesby, epidemiologist Jennifer B. Nuzzo, and physician Tara O'Toole.

Here is the riveting conclusion:

> Experience has shown that communities faced with epidemics or other adverse events respond best and with the least anxiety when the **normal social functioning of the community is least disrupted**. Strong political and public health leadership to provide reassurance and to ensure that needed medical care services are provided are critical elements. If either is seen to be less than optimal, **a manageable epidemic could move toward catastrophe**.

Below we provide a full version of the article. It should help us all to better manage epidemics in the future.

* * *

272 Inglesby, Thomas V., Jennifer B. Nuzzo, Tara O'Toole, and D.A. Henderson. 2006. "Disease Mitigation Measures in the Control of Pandemic Influenza." *Biosecurity and Bioterrorism*, 4(4): 366-375.

## DISEASE MITIGATION MEASURES IN THE CONTROL OF PANDEMIC INFLUENZA[273]

ABSTRACT: The threat of an influenza pandemic has alarmed countries around the globe and given rise to an intense interest in disease mitigation measures. This article reviews what is known about the effectiveness and practical feasibility of a range of actions that might be taken in attempts to lessen the number of cases and deaths resulting from an influenza pandemic. The article also discusses potential adverse second and third order effects of mitigation actions that decision makers must take into account. Finally, the article summarizes the authors' judgments of the likely effectiveness and likely adverse consequences of the range of disease mitigation measures and suggests priorities and practical actions to be taken.

---

The threat of an influenza pandemic, especially one caused by some variant of the highly pathogenic H5N1 avian strains, has alarmed countries around the world. There is universal agreement that the key to influenza prevention is vaccination, and both funds and research are now being expended in pursuit of an effective vaccine. However, producing a satisfactory vaccine will take at least 6 months after a new strain emerges that is demonstrably capable of causing a pandemic. Antiviral drugs offer hope of preventing some cases and possibly diminishing the severity of the disease if they are given within 24–48 hours after onset of symptoms. But supplies of these drugs are limited, the

273 Inglesby, Thomas V., Jennifer B. Nuzzo, Tara O'Toole, and D.A. Henderson. 2006. "Disease Mitigation Measures in the Control of Pandemic Influenza." *Biosecurity and Bioterrorism*, 4(4).

rapid development of virus resistance to the drugs is feared, and they are costly. Accordingly, there has been interest in a range of disease mitigation measures. Possible measures that have been proposed include: isolation of sick people in hospital or at home, use of antiviral medications, handwashing and respiratory etiquette, large-scale or home quarantine of people believed to have been exposed, travel restrictions, prohibition of social gatherings, school closures, maintaining personal distance, and the use of masks. Thus, we must ask whether any or all of the proposed measures are epidemiologically sound, logistically feasible, and politically viable. It is also critically important to consider possible secondary social and economic impacts of various mitigation measures.

Over the years, various combinations of these measures have been used under epidemic and pandemic circumstances in attempts to control the spread of influenza. However, there are few studies that shed light on the relative effectiveness of these measures. A historical review of communities in the U.S. during the 1918 influenza pandemic identified only two that escaped serious mortality and morbidity. Both communities had completely cut themselves off for months from the outside world. One was a remote town in the Colorado mountains, and the other was a naval training station on an island in San Francisco Bay.[274] Obviously, this is not a strategy of general utility. Other studies have suggested that, except in the most extreme applications, disease mitigation measures have not had a significant impact on altering the

---

274 Markel Howard, Alexandra M. Stern, J. Alexander Navarro, Joseph R Michalsen, Arnold S Monto & Cleto DiGiovanni. 2006. "A Historical Assessment of Nonpharmaceutical Disease Mitigation Measures Employed by Selected Communities During the Second Wave of the 1918–1920 Influenza Pandemic." *Emerging Infectious Diseases*, 12(12): 1961-1964.

course of an influenza pandemic.[275]

A number of mitigation measures that are now being considered could have a serious impact on the ability of the health system to deliver adequate care and could have potentially adverse consequences for the provision of essential services. Many could result in significant disruption of the social functioning of communities and result in possibly serious economic problems. Such negative consequences might be worth chancing if there were compelling evidence or reason to believe they would seriously diminish the consequences or spread of a pandemic. However, few analyses have been produced that weigh the hoped-for efficacy of such measures against the potential impacts of large-scale or long-term implementation of these measures.

## EPIDEMIOLOGIC EXPECTATIONS

Historically, it has been all but impossible to prevent influenza from being imported into a country or political jurisdiction, and there has been little evidence that any particular disease mitigation measure has significantly slowed the spread of flu. The clinical and epidemiologic characteristics of influenza explain why:

The influenza virus is known to spread rapidly from one person to the next, with a second generation of patients occurring within 2–4 days following exposure.[276]

---

275 World Health Organization Writing Group. 2006. "Non-Pharmaceutical Public Health Interventions for Pandemic Influenza, National and Community Measures." *Emerging Infectious Diseases*, 12:88–94; Oshitani, Hitoshi. 2006. "Potential benefits and limitations of various strategies to mitigate the impact of an influenza pandemic." *Journal of InfectION Chemotherapy,* 12(4): 167–171.

276 Toner, Eric. 2006. "Do public health and infection control measures prevent the spread of flu?" *Biosecurity and Bioterrorism*, 4(1): 84–86.

People infected with influenza may shed virus for 1–2 days before becoming symptomatic.[277]

Some flu-infected individuals may be asymptomatic and so would not be recognized as being infected. In seasonal flu outbreaks, this group may represent a significant proportion of infected people.[278] Asymptomatic individuals infected with flu have been shown to shed virus, although the extent to which these individuals transmit infection to others is not known.[279]

Many patients who are symptomatic are not readily diagnosed because their symptoms differ little from individuals with other respiratory illnesses or allergies.

## PANDEMIC PLANNING PREMISES

A new pandemic strain can be expected to spread rapidly and widely, but it is not likely to be constantly present in any given area. In both 1918 and 1957, there were some outbreaks in the U.S. of disease in the late spring, but the outbreaks were geographically limited. This has

---

277 Davis, Dorland J, Robert N. Philip, Joseph A. Bell, John E. Bogel and Dinniemaud V. Jensen. 1961. "Epidemiologic Studies on Influenza in Familial and General Population Groups.1951–1956. III. Laboratory Observations." *American Journal of Epidemiology,* 73(2): 138–147.

278 Bridges, Carolyn Buxton, Matthew J. Kuehnert and Caroline B. Hall. 2003. "Transmission of Influenza: Implications for Control in Health Care Settings." *Clinical Infectious Diseases*, 37(8):1094–1101; Foy HM, Cooney MK, Allan ID, Albrecht JK. 1987. "Influenza B in households: virus shedding without symptoms or antibody response." *American Journal of Epidemiology*, 126(3): 506–515.

279 Hayden FG, Fritz R, Lobo MC, Alvord W, Strober W, Straus SE. 1998. "Local and systemic cytokine responses during experimental human influenza A virus infection. Relation to symptom formation and host defense." *The Journal of Clinical Investigation*, 101(3): 643–649.

been referred to as the "first wave" of the pandemic. There were very few cases in the summer, but in the autumn a major pandemic wave of disease swept across the country during a 3–4 month period—the so-called "second wave." This was followed by a comparatively quiescent period, and then a "third wave" occurred the following spring. Subsequently, the new strain in each of these pandemics displaced the then-currently circulating strains and continued to recur every 2–3 years as seasonal flu, although it caused fewer serious illnesses.[280] For planning purposes, the U.S. Department of Health and Human Services (HHS) and the White House Homeland Security Council (HSC) make the assumption that the expected attack rate in the next influenza pandemic would be comparable to the other 20th century pandemics—that is, about 25–30% of the population would become ill.[281] It is also assumed that the virus's ability to spread rapidly and widely would be comparable to past pandemics and that the duration of the outbreak in any given community would be about 8 weeks. While government planners estimate that as much as 30% of the U.S. population would fall sick from the next pandemic, any given community would see those illnesses spaced over a period of at least 8 weeks, not all occurring at one time.[282] Since the average duration of illness would be expected to be about 10 days, only a subset of flu victims in any

---

280 Institute of Medicine. 2004. *The Threat of Pandemic Influenza: Are We Ready?* Washington, DC: Institute of Medicine of the National Academies.

281 U.S. Department of Health and Human Services. 2005. "HHS Pandemic Influenza Plan." Washington, DC: *U.S. Department of Health and Human Services*, November; White House Homeland Security Council. 2006. "National Strategy for Pandemic Influenza: Implementation Plan." Washington, DC: White House Homeland Security Council.

282 Ibid.

community would be ill at once. Given this, even in the peak weeks of a pandemic it would seem reasonable to expect that no more than 10% of a community's population would be ill at any time.

The HHS and HSC documents assume that, in the worst case, the case-fatality ratio would be equal to that of 1918 (about 2.5%).[283] Such data as are available from the past 300 years show the 1918 influenza pandemic was, by far, the most lethal.

To date, the current H5N1 influenza case-fatality ratios have been 50% or more. H5N1 infection has been clinically more severe, and many patients have exhibited symptoms that differ from those caused by other influenza strains.[284] So far, the virus has exhibited little ability to spread from human to human. It has been widely assumed that if the current avian strain of virus did transform into one that is more readily transmissible, the virus would assume characteristics and case-fatality rates more closely resembling previous pandemic strains. A range of possible measures for containing the spread of influenza during a pandemic are set forth in HHS's Pandemic Influenza Plan and HSC's *National Strategy for Pandemic Influenza: Implementation Plan.*[285] Both documents outline possible actions that might be taken during a pandemic to minimize transmission and control the spread of infection.

---

283 White House Homeland Security Council (2006).

284 World Health Organization. 2006. "Epidemiology of WHO-confirmed human cases of avian A(H5N1) infection." *Weekly Epidemiol Record,* June 30, 81(26): 249–260; Tran, Tinh Hien, Thanh Liem Nguyen, Thi Dung Nguyen, Thi San Luong, Phuong Mai Pham et al. 2004. "Avian influenza A (H5N1) in 10 patients in Vietnam." *New England Journal of Medicine,* March 18, 350(12): 1179–1188.

285 U.S. Department of Health and Human Services (2005); White House Homeland Security Council (2006).

Disease mitigation measures are presented as a series of options, but the criteria for pursuing any particular measure are not articulated nor are operational details provided regarding how these measures should be implemented.

It has been recognized that most actions taken to counter pandemic influenza will have to be undertaken by local governments, given that the epidemic response capacity of the federal government is limited.[286] This is reflected in HHS Secretary Michael Leavitt's statement at a February 2006 State and Local Pandemic Preparedness Meeting: "Any community that fails to prepare [for an influenza pandemic] with the idea that somehow, in the end, the federal government will be able to rescue them will be tragically wrong."[287] But a recent review of the current pandemic influenza plans of 49 states reveals that few explicitly discuss implementing community mitigation strategies.[288] The authors of the review attribute this lack of planning for influenza in part to "weak central (federal) direction and the lack of key epidemiological data."[289] One of the better developed plans is that of the New York City Department of Health and Mental Hygiene, whose staff considered the use of disease mitigation measures but decided to incorporate few

---

286 Barbera, Joseph, Anthony Macintyre, Craig DeAtley, Larry Gostin, Tom Inglesby et al. 2001. "Large-scale quarantine following biological terrorism in the United States: scientific examination, logistic and legal limits, and possible consequences." *JAMA,* 286(21): 2711–2717.

287 U.S. Department of Health and Human Services. 2006. *State of Maryland Summit on Influenza Pandemic, February 26, 2006; Baltimore, Maryland.*

288 Holmberg, Scott D., Christine M. Layton, George S. Ghneim, and Diane K. Wagener. 2006. "State plans for containment of pandemic influenza." *Emerging Infectious Diseases*, 12(9): 1414–1417.

289 Ibid.

of the measures now described in federal plans.[290]

A fundamental premise of disease mitigation that has been advanced by some in the policymaking community is that a less intense but more prolonged pandemic may be easier for society to bear, but this is speculative.[291]

## CLARIFICATION OF TERMS

There is widespread confusion about the terms used to describe measures for controlling disease spread. The principal confusion is between use of the words quarantine and isolation. Isolation properly refers only to the confinement of symptomatic patients in the hospital (or at home) so that they will not infect others. Quarantine has traditionally been defined as the separation from circulation in the community of asymptomatic people who may have been exposed to infection and might—or might not—become ill. Home quarantine refers to voluntary confinement of known contacts of influenza cases in their own homes. Large-scale quarantine typically refers to confinement of large groups of possibly infected people—for example, all passengers on an airplane, or the residents of an apartment building or an entire city—for periods of days to weeks.

In recent years the term social distancing has come into use. Social distancing has been used to refer to a range of measures that might serve to reduce contact between people. These may include closing

---

290 New York City Department of Health and Mental Hygiene. 2006. "NYC DOHMH pandemic influenza preparedness and response plan." *New York City Department of Health and Mental Hygiene*, July.

291 Cetron M. 2006. *Presentation at CDC Meeting on Community Mitigation Strategies for Pandemic Influenza Consultants Meeting, Atlanta, Georgia, June 14, 2006.*

schools or prohibiting large gatherings, such as church services and sporting events. Others have used the term to refer to actions taken to increase the distance of individuals from each other at the work site or in other locations—for example, substituting phone calls for face-to-face meetings or avoiding hand-shaking. The term has come to describe fundamentally different approaches to disease mitigation. This document will refer only to specific interventions rather than to the catch-all term social distancing.

## EVALUATION OF DISEASE MITIGATION MEASURES

**Epidemiologic Assessment: Do available data or experience suggest the measure will work?**

It is difficult to evaluate the effectiveness of specific measures to control disease spread in epidemiologic terms because of the complex interrelationships between individuals and groups and the individual biological differences in response to influenza. Some historical studies have tried to evaluate the efficacy of specific influenza containment efforts, and, although they are informative, the relative paucity of such studies and the differences between past historical moments and the present limit the conclusions that can be drawn.[292]

Recently, a number of mathematical models have examined various

292 World Health Organization Writing Group (2006).

combinations of disease mitigation measures for pandemic influenza.[293] Such models consist of computer simulations of disease outbreaks that are developed from very limited data regarding the epidemiological and biological characteristics of influenza and a series of assumptions about the likely compliance of the population, the feasibility of applying various interventions, and so on. The predictions provided by such models can vary widely depending on the assumptions that are made in their construction.

What the computer models cannot incorporate is the effects that various mitigation strategies might have on the behavior of the population and the consequent course of the epidemic. There is simply too little experience to predict how a 21st century population would respond, for example, to the closure of all schools for periods of many weeks to months, or to the cancellation of all gatherings of more than 1,000 persons. Would these closures serve to decrease contacts between people and so retard the spread of the epidemic? Or would those affected spend more time in malls, in fast-food restaurants, and in other social settings that might result in more contacts and more rapid spread of influenza?

No model, no matter how accurate its epidemiologic assumptions, can illuminate or predict the secondary and tertiary effects of particular disease mitigation measures. Nor, for example, can it assess

---

293 Germann Timothy C., Kai Kadau, Ira M. Longini Jr., and Catherine A. Macken. 2006. "Mitigation strategies for pandemic influenza in the United States." *Proceedings of the National Academy of Sciences USA,* April 11, 103(15): 5935–5940; Hollingsworth TD, Ferguson NM, Anderson RM. 2006. "Will travel restrictions control the international spread of pandemic influenza?" *Nature Medicine*, 12(5): 497–499. Ferguson, Neil M, Derek A.T. Cummings, Christophe Fraser, James C. Cajka, Philip C. Cooley & Donald S. Burke. 2006. "Measures for mitigating an influenza pandemic." *Nature,* 442(7101): 448–452.

the potential effects of high absentee rates resulting from home or regional quarantine on the functioning integrity of essential services, such as hospital care or provision of food and electrical service to the community. If particular measures are applied for many weeks or months, the long-term or cumulative second and third order effects could be devastating socially and economically. In brief, models can play a contributory role in thinking through possible mitigation measures, but they cannot be more than an ancillary aid in deciding policy.

**Logistical Assessment: Is the disease mitigation measure feasible?** Many communitywide disease mitigation measures would be intrinsically difficult to implement. Consideration must be given to the resources required for implementation, to the mechanisms needed to persuade the public to comply (or to compel the public, if the measures are mandatory), and to the length of time that they would need to be applied. Potential disease mitigation measures presumably would have to be maintained for the duration of the epidemic in a community—a predicted period of 8 or more weeks—or, perhaps, in the country as a whole—as long as 8 months.[294]

Recent experiences in endeavoring to quarantine large numbers of people during the 2003 SARS outbreaks illustrate why feasibility must be a central consideration. Canadian health officials implemented a voluntary home quarantine in Toronto, where an estimated 30,000 people who came in contact with SARS cases (fewer than 500 actual cases in all) were asked to stay home until it became clear that they

294 Cetron (2006).

were not infected.[295] Although the efficacy of the home quarantine in Toronto is not clear, the public health resources needed to implement this policy were prodigious, as it was necessary not only to persuade each family of the rationale of the measures and inform them how to comply but also to arrange to provide food and other support services. As a result of this and other experiences, medical authorities have expressed doubts about the efficacy and feasibility of large-scale and home quarantines.[296]

**Social, Economic, and Political Assessment: What are the possible unintended adverse societal consequences?**

Disease mitigation measures, however well intentioned, have potential social, economic, and political consequences that need to be fully considered by political leaders as well as health officials. Closing schools is an example. Some have suggested closure might be recommended for as long as a pandemic persists in a single community (perhaps 8 weeks) or for as long as a pandemic persists in the country (as long as 8 months).[297] The rationale for the strategy is to diminish contacts between students and so retard epidemic spread. However, if this strategy were to be successful, other sites where school children gather

---

295 DiGiovanni, Clete, Jerome Conley, Daniel Chiu, and Jason Zaborski. 2004. "Factors influencing compliance with quarantine in Toronto during the 2003 SARS outbreak." *Biosecurity and Bioterrorism*, 2(4): 265–272.

296 Barbera et al. (2001); U.S. Centers for Disease Control and Prevention. 2003. "Efficiency of quarantine during an epidemic of Severe Acute Respiratory Syndrome—Beijing, China, 2003." *Morbidity and Mortality Weekly Report*, 52(43): 1037–1040; Schabas R. 2003. "SARS: Prudence, not panic." *CMAJ*, 168(11): 1432–1434.

297 Cetron (2006).

would also have to be closed: daycare centers, cinemas, churches, fast-food stores, malls, and athletic arenas. Many parents would need to stay home from work to care for children, which could result in high rates of absenteeism that could stress critical services, including health care. School closures also raise the question of whether certain segments of society would be forced to bear an unfair share of the disease control burden. A significant proportion of children in lower-income families rely on school feeding programs for basic nutrition.

Political leaders need to understand the likely benefits and the potential consequences of disease mitigation measures, including the possible loss of critical civic services and the possible loss of confidence in government to manage the crisis.

## POTENTIAL DISEASE CONTROL MEASURES: BENEFITS AND CONSEQUENCES

### Large-Scale Community Vaccination

Vaccines are the best mechanism for preventing influenza infection and spread in the community and for protecting healthcare workers caring for those who do become ill. Once an influenza strain capable of sustained human-to-human transmission emerges, a vaccine specific to the pandemic strain will need to be made. It is expected that it will be at least 6 months after the emergence of the pandemic strain before the initial supplies of vaccine can be produced. Current vaccine manufacturing techniques and limitations on vaccine production constrain the total amount of vaccine that can be manufactured. Special efforts are being made to increase this capacity, but under current conditions, according to the National Strategy for Pandemic Influenza, it will be as much as 5 years (i.e., 2011) before domestic vaccine production capacity is in place to create enough vaccine for the entire U.S. population within 6 months of the start of a pandemic.[298]

**Isolation of Sick People in Hospitals**

Beyond widespread vaccination, isolating symptomatic influenza patients, either at home or in the hospital, is probably the most important measure that could be taken to reduce the transmission and slow the spread of illness within a community. The sickest (and presumably most contagious) patients are most likely to seek hospital care. The critical importance of hospitals in providing health care during a pandemic cannot be overstated and has been addressed by a number of sources.[299]

In an influenza epidemic, hospitals will face several key challenges. First, hospitals must protect their own staffs from infection and avoid becoming "amplifiers" of disease. Historically, hospitals have often accelerated the spread of contagious disease because of the presence of highly contagious patients and their close proximity to the medical

---

298 White House Homeland Security Council (2006); Roos, Robert. 2006. "Glaxo says its H5N1 vaccine works at low dose." *CIDRAP News*, July 26.

299 Franco, Crystal, Eric Toner, Richard Walhorn, Beth Maldin, Tara O'Toole, and Tomas V. Inglesby. 2006. "Systemic collapse: medical care in the aftermath of hurricane Katrina." *Biosecurity and Bioterrorism*, 4(2): 135–146; Toner, Eric, Richard Waldhorn, Beth Maldin, et al. 2006. "Hospital preparedness for pandemic influenza." *Biosecurity and Bioterrorism*, 4(2): 207–217. American College of Physicians. 2006. "The health care response to pandemic influenza." *Annals of Internal Medicine*, 145(2):135–137. Hick, John L., Dan Hanfling, Jonathan L. Burstein, Craig DeAtley, Donna Barbisch et al. 2004. "Health care facility and community measures for patient care surge capacity." *Annals of Emergency Medicine*, 44(3): 253–261; Rubinson, Lewis, Jennifer B. Nuzzo, Daniel S. Talmor, Tara O'Toole, Bradley R. Kramer, and Thomas V. Inglesby. 2005. "Augmentation of hospital critical care capacity after bioterrorist attacks or epidemics: recommendations of the Working Group on Emergency Mass Critical Care." *Critical Care Medicine*, 33(10): 2393–2403.

staff who care for them and to other patients who are ill and vulnerable to infection.[300] Modern hospitals are not designed to accommodate large numbers of highly contagious patients, and special measures, including cohorting of patients, adjustments to HVAC systems, and use of personal protective gear, will need to be made to protect healthcare workers and patients from infection. Second, hospitals must establish strategies for coping with what will presumably be a large and relatively sustained surge in demand for medical care. At present, hospitals have little capacity to meet such demands.[301] Hospital care will be needed not only for those who are ill with influenza itself but also for patients with chronic conditions made critical by acute influenza infection. Accommodating the increased demand for hospital care will require coordination and collaboration between hospitals in a given region and among hospital leaders, public health authorities, and elected officials. Some jurisdictions have taken steps to establish the organizational framework, communication networks, and operational principles needed to do this, but most have not.[302] It is noteworthy that, in spite of the predominant role that hospitals must play in pandemic response, the federal allocations for pandemic flu preparedness have included little financial support either for regional medical care planning or for

300 Chiarello, Linda A., and Michael L. Tapper. 2004. "Healthcare settings as amplifiers of infectious disease." *Emerging Infectious Diseases*, 10(11): 2048–2049.

301 Toner et al. (2006); Rubinson et al. (2005); Bartlett, John G. 2006. "Planning for avian influenza." *Annals of Internal Medicine*, 145(2): 141–144.

302 Hick et al. (2004).

the hospitals themselves.[303]

In 1918–19, even the best-equipped hospitals had little to offer flu victims. Today, however, although modern medicine offers limited remedies for influenza, the availability of oxygen, ventilators, antibiotics, and parenteral fluids could make a critical difference in surviving flu, especially among those with underlying chronic disease.

It has been suggested that alternative care sites, such as gymnasiums and armories, could lessen the demand on hospitals.[304] In 1918, such alternative care facilities were set up in many cities. However, patients housed in alternative sites received little more than food and water. Such sites realistically would represent alternatives to home care, not hospital care, given the practical problems of safely managing services such as respiratory support, intravenous medication, oxygen, and the like outside of a hospital setting. A major challenge for all authorities charged with managing a pandemic will be how to allot scarce, possibly life-saving medical resources and how to maintain hospitals' capacity to care for critically ill flu victims while continuing to provide other essential medical services.

### Home Isolation of Sick People

In light of the expected shortages of medical beds and personnel, home isolation of non-critically ill influenza patients would be necessary in

---

303 Levi, Jeffrey, and Thomas Inglesby. 2006. "Working Group on Pandemic Influenza Preparedness: joint statement in response to Department of Health and Human Services Pandemic Influenza Plan." *Clinical Infectious Diseases*, 42(1): 92–94.

304 U.S. Department of Health and Human Services (2005); National Association of County and City Health Officials. 2006. "Local Health Department Guide to Pandemic Influenza Planning." Washington, DC: NACCHO.

a major pandemic. A policy that persuades sick individuals to voluntarily stay at home unless they are critically ill would allow hospitals to focus efforts on those most seriously threatened.

There are a number of logistical considerations that could prevent people from being able to remain isolated in their homes. Special measures would be needed to provide basic medical and food supplies, perhaps through the use of neighborhood volunteers and supplemented by communication by phone or internet. It may not be easy to persuade those without paid sick leave (some 59 million persons) to absent themselves from work, unless employers address this problem directly.[305] A recent review of state pandemic influenza plans found that only one-third of the 49 states examined have explicit plans to encourage voluntary home isolation.[306]

### Use of Antiviral Medications

Antiviral drugs for influenza are available in limited quantities. Data on how antivirals might perform in the prevention or treatment of the H5N1 strain are scant. Prominent authorities think the likelihood of "quenching" an emergent pandemic strain through the rapid, regionwide use of antivirals is low because of technical and logistical difficulties, even if the pandemic strain proves to be sensitive to such drugs.[307] Several countries have recommended that the top priority for

---

305 Lovell, Vicky. 2003. *No Time to Be Sick: Why Everyone Suffers When Workers Don't Have Paid Sick Leave.* Washington, DC: Institute for Women's Policy Research; December.

306 Holmberg et al. (2006).

307 Lancet Editorial. 2006. "A reappraisal of H5N1 avian influenza." *Lancet,* May 13; 367(9522): 1550.

antivirals is to treat the ill.[308] If antivirals were to be used for prevention, it would imply the need for much longer administration of the drug to cover the period of a community epidemic. Specifically, using oseltamivir as the most available example, the quantity of antivirals used to prevent infection in a single healthcare worker during an 8–10-week epidemic period would serve to treat an estimated 5 to 7 patients (assumes prophylaxis with 75 mg, twice daily, for 8–10 weeks versus treatment with 150 mg, twice daily, for 5 days).[309]

Moreover, available data indicate that antiviral treatment is effective only if antivirals are given within 24–48 hours after onset of initial symptoms.[310] Some authorities doubt the feasibility of administering the drugs soon enough to make a difference during a pandemic.[311] Because of this concern, at least one Canadian teaching hospital is planning to use all its antiviral stocks for prophylaxis of healthcare workers.[312] The European Union, on the other hand, decided not to stockpile any antiviral medicines, although some European countries

---

308 U.K. Health Departments. 2005. "Pandemic Flu: Influenza Pandemic Contingency Plan." *UK Health Department*, October; Public Health Agency of Canada. 2004. "Canadian Pandemic Influenza Plan." *Public Health Agency of Canada*, February.

309 Ward, Penelope, Ian Small, James Smith, Pia Suter, and Regina Dutkowski. 2005. "Oseltamivir (Tamiflu) and its potential for use in the event of an influenza pandemic." *The Journal of Antimicrobial Chemotherapy,* 55 (Suppl 1):i5–i21.

310 Roche Pharmaceuticals. "Product Information: Tamiflu® capsules and for oral suspension, oseltamivir phosphate." *Roche Pharmaceuticals.*

311 Holmberg et al. (2006); Bartlett (2006); Hayden FG. 2004. "Pandemic influenza: is an antiviral response realistic?" *The Pediatric Infectious Disease Journal*, 23(11 Suppl):S262–S269.

312 Branswell H. T.O. 2006. hospitals to stockpile drug. *Canadian Press News Service*, May 31.

have done so.[313]

The effectiveness and optimal use of antivirals remain uncertain because of several factors: the propensity of the influenza virus to mutate, thus increasing the possibility that resistance could develop; the quantities of antivirals required for prophylaxis; and the logistical challenges involved in providing sufficiently rapid treatment. Contextual variables that cannot be predicted ahead of time—such as the quantity of medicines available and the development of resistance—will probably determine antiviral strategy.

**Hand-Washing and Respiratory Etiquette**

The influenza virus actually survives on the hands for less than 5 minutes, but regular hand-washing is a commonsense action that should be widely followed.[314] It has been shown to reduce the transmission of respiratory illness in a military trainee setting, although there are no data to demonstrate that hand-washing deters the spread of influenza within a community.[315]

General respiratory hygiene, such as covering one's mouth when coughing and using disposable paper tissues, is widely believed to be of some value in diminishing spread, even though there is no hard evidence that this is so.

313 Mounier-Jack, Sandra, and Richard J. Coker. 2006. "How prepared is Europe for pandemic influenza? Analysis of national plans." *Lancet,* April 29, 367(9520): 1405–1411.

314 Toner (2006).

315 Ryan, Margaret A.K., Rebecca S. Christian, and Julie Wohlrabe. 2001. "Handwashing and respiratory illness among young adults in military training." *American Journal of Preventive Medicine,* 21(2): 79–83.

## Large-Scale Quarantine Measures

There are no historical observations or scientific studies that support the confinement by quarantine of groups of possibly infected people for extended periods in order to slow the spread of influenza. A World Health Organization (WHO) Writing Group, after reviewing the literature and considering contemporary international experience, concluded that "forced isolation and quarantine are ineffective and impractical."[316] Despite this recommendation by experts, mandatory large-scale quarantine continues to be considered as an option by some authorities and government officials.[317]

The interest in quarantine reflects the views and conditions prevalent more than 50 years ago, when much less was known about the epidemiology of infectious diseases and when there was far less international and domestic travel in a less densely populated world. It is difficult to identify circumstances in the past half-century when large-scale quarantine has been effectively used in the control of any disease. The negative consequences of large-scale quarantine are so extreme (forced confinement of sick people with the well; complete restriction of movement of large populations; difficulty in getting critical supplies, medicines, and food to people inside the quarantine zone) that this mitigation measure should be eliminated from serious consideration.

## Home Quarantine

Voluntary home quarantine would be requested of individuals who are asymptomatic but who have had substantial contact with a person who

---

316 World Health Organization Writing Group (2006).

317 Lovell (2003); Mounier-Jack (2006).

has influenza—primarily household members. The aim of voluntary home quarantine is to keep possibly contagious, but still asymptomatic, people out of circulation. This sounds logical, but this measure raises significant practical and ethical issues.

If implemented on a communitywide scale, logistical requirements related to ensuring that quarantined households across a community had appropriate care and support would be necessary. How compliant the public might be is uncertain. Parents would presumably be willing to stay home and care for sick children, but it is not known, for example, whether college students would agree to be interned with infected dorm-mates.

Even if home quarantine were generally acceptable to the community, individuals may not have the economic resources to stay at home. Few employers currently have provisions for paid absence unless the workers themselves are ill. For those who are hourly workers or who are self-employed, the potential loss of wages as a result of having to stay home simply because an individual had had contact with sick people might not be acceptable or feasible.

Home quarantine also raises ethical questions. Implementation of home quarantine could result in healthy, uninfected people being placed at risk of infection from sick household members. Practices to reduce the chance of transmission (hand-washing, maintaining a distance of 3 feet from infected people, etc.) could be recommended, but a policy imposing home quarantine would preclude, for example, sending healthy children to stay with relatives when a family member becomes ill. Such a policy would also be particularly hard on and dangerous to people living in close quarters, where the risk of infection would be heightened.

**Travel Restrictions**

Travel restrictions, such as closing airports and screening travelers at borders, have historically been ineffective. The World Health Organization Writing Group concluded that "screening and quarantining entering travelers at international borders did not substantially delay virus introduction in past pandemics... and will likely be even less effective in the modern era."[318]

Similar conclusions were reached by public health authorities involved in the international efforts to control SARS. Canadian health authorities report that "available screening measures for SARS were limited in their effectiveness in detecting SARS among inbound or outbound passengers from SARS-affected areas."[319] A review by a WHO Working Group on SARS also concluded that "entry screening of travelers through health declarations or thermal scanning at international borders had little documented effect on detecting SARS cases."[320]

The authors have concluded in a previous analysis that screening individuals on domestic interstate flights for symptoms of flu, as has been proposed in revisions to the Federal Quarantine Rule (42 CFR Parts 70 and 71), would not be effective and would have serious adverse

---

318 World Health Organization Writing Group (2006).

319 St. John, Ronald K., Arlene King, Dick de Jong, Margaret Bodie-Collins, Susan G. Squires, and Theresa W.S. Tam. 2005. "Border screening for SARS." *Emerging Infectious Diseases*, 11(1): 6–10.

320 Bell, David M., and World Health Organization Working Group on Prevention of International and Community Transmission of SARS. 2004. "Public health interventions and SARS spread, 2003." *Emerging Infectious Diseases*, 10(11): 1900–1906.

consequences.[321]

It is reasonable to assume that the economic costs of shutting down air or train travel would be very high, and the societal costs involved in interrupting all air or train travel would be extreme. Shutting down public transportation for an extended period is not an option in many cities. In New York City, an average of 4.7 million people ride the subway each weekday; the Los Angeles Metro averages 1.3 million riders daily.[322]

**Prohibition of Social Gatherings**

During seasonal influenza epidemics, public events with an expected large attendance have sometimes been cancelled or postponed, the rationale being to decrease the number of contacts with those who might be contagious. There are, however, no certain indications that these actions have had any definitive effect on the severity or duration of an epidemic. Were consideration to be given to doing this on a more extensive scale and for an extended period, questions immediately arise as to how many such events would be affected. There are many social gatherings that involve close contacts among people, and this prohibition might include church services, athletic events, perhaps

---

321 Nuzzo, Jennifer B., Donald A. HendersonTara O'Toole, and Thomas V. Inglesby. 2006. "Comments from the Center for Biosecurity of UPMC on proposed revisions to federal quarantine rules." *Biosecurity and Bioterrorism*, 4(2): 204–206; U.S. National Archives Federal Register. "Control of Communicable Disease, Federal Register 229" (proposed November 30, 2005) (to be codified at 42 C.F.R. pts. 70, 71).

322NYC Metropolitan Transit Authority. "Subway Facts." *New York City Metropolitan Transit Authority*; LA Metropolitan Transportation Authority. "Bus Ridership Estimates." *Los Angeles County Metropolitan Transportation Authority.*

all meetings of more than 100 people. It might mean closing theaters, restaurants, malls, large stores, and bars. Implementing such measures would have seriously disruptive consequences for a community if extended through the 8-week period of an epidemic in a municipal area, let alone if it were to be extended through the nation's experience with a pandemic (perhaps 8 months).[323] In the event of a pandemic, attendance at public events or social gatherings could well decrease because people were fearful of becoming infected, and some events might be cancelled because of local concerns. But a policy calling for community wide cancellation of public events seems inadvisable.

**School Closures**

In previous influenza epidemics, the impact of school closings on illness rates has been mixed.[324] A study from Israel reported a decrease in respiratory infections after a 2-week teacher strike, but the decrease was only evident for a single day.[325] On the other hand, when schools closed for a winter holiday during the 1918 pandemic in Chicago, "more influenza cases developed among pupils... than when schools were in session."[326]

Schools are often closed for 1–2 weeks early in the development of

---

323 DiGiovanni (2004).

324 World Health Organization Writing Group (2006).

325 Heymann, Anthony, Gabriel Chodick, Brian Reichman, Ehud Kokia, and Joseph Laufer. 2004. "Influence of school closure on the incidence of viral respiratory diseases among children and on health care utilization." *The Pediatric Infectious Disease Journal*, 23(7): 675–677.

326 World Health Organization Writing Group (2006); Jordan, EO. 1919. "Influenza in three Chicago groups." *The Journal of Infectious Diseases*, 25: 74–95.

seasonal community outbreaks of influenza primarily because of high absentee rates, especially in elementary schools, and because of illness among teachers. This would seem reasonable on practical grounds. However, to close schools for longer periods is not only impracticable but carries the possibility of a serious adverse outcome. For example, for working parents, school serves as a form of day care and, in some areas, a source of nutritional meals for children from lower-income families. In 2005, some 29.5 million children were fed through the National School Lunch Program; 9.3 million children received meals as part of the School Breakfast Program.[327] A portion of America's workforce would be unable to go to work as long as children were out of schools. Heightened absentee rates could cripple essential service industries. Teachers might not be paid and a great many hourly workers (mall and fast-food employees; school janitorial, security, and kitchen staff; bus drivers) would face particular financial hardship.

### Maintaining Personal Distance

It has been recommended that individuals maintain a distance of 3 feet or more during a pandemic so as to diminish the number of contacts with people who may be infected.[328] The efficacy of this measure is unknown. It is typically assumed that transmission of droplet-spread diseases, such as influenza, is limited to "close contacts"—that is,

327 U.S. Department of Agriculture. 2006. "Food and Nutrition Service Data." *U.S. Department of Agriculture.*

328 U.S. Department of Health and Human Services (2005); U.S. Department of Health and Human Services, Federal Occupational Health. 2006. "Top 10 Tips for Pandemic Preparedness and Prevention."

being within 3–6 feet of an infected person.[329] Keeping a space of 3 feet between individuals might be possible in some work environments, but it is difficult to imagine how bus, rail, or air travelers could stay 3 feet apart from each other throughout an epidemic. And such a recommendation would greatly complicate normal daily tasks like grocery shopping, banking, and the like.

**Use of Masks and Personal Protective Equipment**

Masks and other personal protective equipment (PPE) are essential for controlling transmission of influenza in hospitals. For people who work in hospitals, current CDC guidelines for influenza infection control recommend droplet precautions, including the use of surgical masks. But HHS planning guidelines also rightly acknowledge that the uncertainties regarding the potential of virus transmission at the start of a new pandemic would recommend that airborne precautions be used in hospitals—that is, N95 masks (already in short supply) or powered air purifying respirators (PAPRs).[330] Patients would be advised to wear surgical masks to diminish the number of infectious respiratory particles being dispersed into the air, thereby diminishing the likelihood of further spread.[331]

In Asia during the SARS period, many people in the affected

---

329 Toner (2006).

330 U.S. Department of Health and Human Services (2005); Foy, H.M., M.K. Cooney, I.D. Allan, and J.K. Albrecht. 1987. "Influenza B in households: virus shedding without symptoms or antibody response." *American Journal of Epidemiology*, 126(3): 506–515.

331 Grow, Robert W., and Lewis Rubinson. 2003. "The challenge of hospital infection control during a response to bioterrorist attacks." *Biosecurity and Bioterrorism*, 1(3): 215–220.

communities wore surgical masks when in public. But studies have shown that the ordinary surgical mask does little to prevent inhalation of small droplets bearing influenza virus.[332] The pores in the mask become blocked by moisture from breathing, and the airstream simply diverts around the mask. There are few data available to support the efficacy of N95 or surgical masks outside a healthcare setting. N95 masks need to be fit-tested to be efficacious and are uncomfortable to wear for more than an hour or two.[333] More important, the supplies of such masks are too limited to even ensure that hospitals will have necessary reserves.[334]

## COMMUNITY RESPONSE TO A PANDEMIC: A SUMMARY OF POSSIBLE ACTIONS

There is no question but that another influenza pandemic will occur and that every community needs to be prepared for that eventuality. Influenza is unlike any other disease epidemic in the rapidity with which it spreads and, as it emerges, the number of illnesses that it can cause over a period of a few months. It is unpredictable as to when a pandemic might begin. It could be next autumn or it may not be for a number of years. The world has weathered three pandemics during

---

332 Balazy, Anna, Mika Toivola, Atin Adhikari, Satheesh K. Sivasubramani, Tiina reponen, and Sergey A. Grinshpun. 2006. "Do N95 respirators provide 95% protection level against airborne viruses, and how adequate are surgical masks?" *American Journal of Infection Control*, 34(2): 51–57.

333 Grow and Rubinson (2003); U.S. Centers for Disease Control and Prevention. "Interim Recommendations for Infection Control in Health-Care Facilities Caring for Patients with Known or Suspected Avian Influenza." *U.S. Centers for Disease Control and Prevention.*

334 2006. "Six respirator manufacturers warn President Bush of imminent shortage of masks necessary for avian flu pandemic response." *Medical News Today*, June 24.

the past century and will certainly surmount the next one. How much damage the pandemic will cause depends to a large extent on the state of readiness of each community and each metropolitan region and the efficacy and reasonableness of its response. The following is a synopsis of the authors' judgments regarding possible disease mitigation measures.

***Vaccination*.** Vaccination is, by far, the most important preventive measure, but pandemic strain vaccine will not be available for at least the next season. Meanwhile, communitywide use of the seasonal influenza vaccine is desirable, as it is likely that outbreaks of seasonal flu will occur even if there is pandemic influenza.

***Provision for isolation and medical care of influenza patients*.** A Regional Health Care Operations Committee is a priority need to assure collaboration and cooperation across the community (hospitals, medical care providers, Red Cross, law enforcement, media, and others), both for advanced planning and during the epidemic to assure that the large numbers of flu-infected patients can be cared for in hospital, at home, or in special facilities.[335] Special arrangements are needed for expanding surge capacity in hospitals, for support to permit home care of patients, and for the provision of additional volunteer healthcare staff.

***A communication strategy and plans*.** Open and frequent communications with the public are essential. This involves regular press conferences, hot lines, and provision of information through civic

335 Toner et al. (2006).

leaders, churches, schools, and businesses. An important message is to request that all who are ill remain isolated at home or in the hospital but to encourage others to continue to come to work so that essential services can be sustained.

***Closure of schools***. It has been the practice in many communities to close the schools for 10–14 days at the beginning of an epidemic of seasonal flu, primarily because of the number of both teachers and pupils who are absent. This is a reasonable initiative, often expected in many communities, that also serves to demonstrate action on the part of officials. Closing schools for longer periods in hopes of mitigating the epidemic by decreasing contacts among students is not warranted unless all other likely points of assembly are closed (e.g., malls, fast-food restaurants, churches, recreation centers, etc.). Such widespread closures, sustained throughout the pandemic, would almost certainly have serious adverse social and economic effects.

***Hand-washing and respiratory hygiene***. Everyone should be encouraged to wash their hands after coming in contact with people who are ill and to cover their mouths when coughing or sneezing.

***Cancelling or postponing meetings or events involving large numbers of people***. Intuitively, this would appear to be a helpful adjunct to reduce contacts among people and so mitigate the effects of the epidemic. However, individuals normally have a great many contacts throughout the community on a daily basis: shopping in stores, attending church, traveling on public transport, and so on. Recognizing that the spread of influenza is primarily by person-to-person contact, any one individual, even in a large gathering, would have only a limited number of such close encounters with infected people. Thus, cancelling or postponing large meetings would not be likely to have any significant effect on the development of the epidemic. While local concerns may result in the closure of particular events for logical reasons, a policy directing communitywide closure of public events seems inadvisable.

***Quarantine.*** As experience shows, there is no basis for recommending quarantine either of groups or individuals. The problems in implementing such measures are formidable, and secondary effects of absenteeism and community disruption as well as possible adverse consequences, such as loss of public trust in government and stigmatization of quarantined people and groups, are likely to be considerable.

***Screening passengers at borders or closing air or rail hubs***. Experience has shown that these actions are not effective and could have serious adverse consequences; thus, they are not recommended.

***An overriding principle***. Experience has shown that communities faced with epidemics or other adverse events respond best and with the least anxiety when the normal social functioning of the community is least disrupted. Strong political and public health leadership to provide reassurance and to ensure that needed medical care services are provided are critical elements. If either is seen to be less than optimal, a manageable epidemic could move toward catastrophe.

## THE EPISTEMIC BURDEN OF POLITICS

### BY ETHAN YANG

July 20, 2020

Former Secretary of Defense Donald Rumsfield once famously remarked in a press conference that,[336]

> There are known knowns; there are things we know we know. We also know there are known unknowns; that is to say we know there are some things we do not know. But there are also unknown unknowns—the ones we don't know we don't know.

It is highly possible he could have found a better way to articulate his thoughts but nonetheless his statement carried a profound lesson: policymakers face tremendous burdens in understanding what they do and do not know. We trust our leaders in government to make informed decisions on our behalf and a failure to understand the full implications of a policy will adversely affect countless individuals.

Arizona State University Professor Scott Scheall explores the topic of knowledge acquisition in policymaking in his latest book *F.A. Hayek and the Epistemology of Politics: The Curious Task of Economics*.[337] His work serves as an extension and expansion of the thinking espoused by legendary economist Friedrich Hayek. The phrase at the end of the book's title is part of a famous Hayek quote that begins:

---

336 CNN. 2016. "Rumsfeld / Knowns." *YouTube*, March 31.

337 Scheall, Scott. 2020. *F.A. Hayek and the Epistemology of Politics: The Curious Task of Economics*. Routledge.

> The curious task of economics is to demonstrate to men how little they really know about what they imagine they can design.[338]

Hayek was speaking to the vast hubris that permeates the minds of policy experts and decision-makers. Through economic analysis, particularly through the Austrian school of thought, the viewer should understand that society has countless individual needs and desires. That there is a natural order that arises regardless of the will or blessings of a central administrator. That disrupting that order with restrictive, clumsy, and misinformed government policy will only bring unintended consequences.

This is the essence of the rest of Hayek's famous quote as he remarks:

> It may seem absurd that in complex conditions order, and adaptation to the unknown, can be achieved more effectively by decentralizing decisions and that a division of authority will actually extend the possibility of overall order. Yet that decentralization actually leads to more information being taken into account.

This is the topic Scheall explores quite deeply in his aforementioned book, *Political Epistemology*. According to the Oxford Dictionary, epistemology is:

338 Hayek, Friedrich A. "The Fatal Conceit Quotes." *Good Reads.*

> The theory of knowledge, especially with regard to its methods, validity, and scope. Epistemology is the investigation of what distinguishes justified belief from opinion.[339]

How do those in government such as elected officials and bureaucrats know exactly what their constituents want? How do they know truly what is the best course of action in response to a recession or a pandemic? Are they adequately equipped to understand the tradeoffs and consequences of their decisions? For the most part, liberal democracies seem to implicitly acknowledge their epistemic shortcomings.

They understand that market mechanisms like prices, private property, supply and demand, and individual autonomy are far superior to central planning in delivering the needs of society. Although economic and civil freedom is good for many other noble causes like general prosperity and preventing tyranny, they ultimately function as a means to process information about society. Through these market mechanisms, we are able to find solutions to all sorts of knowledge problems such as how to construct a global credit network, or how to leverage supply chains that span the planet to feed billions. These incredibly difficult questions are answered by decentralized and voluntary decision-making.

Scheall's book points out how the political process is simply another means to acquire knowledge to execute decisions, albeit an inferior one. Elected officials are simply surrogates that individuals appointed to wield the power of the state and make decisions on their behalf.

---

339 Lexico. 2020. "Epistemology." *Lexico*.

The political process, voting, town halls, lobbying, debating: these are means in which a single individual, the policymaker, attempts to acquire knowledge that is dispersed throughout society.

Scheall recommends that if we wish to retrieve the best outcomes from government action, we must understand the epistemic burdens of policymakers and come to terms with their limits. He explains what he means by this when he writes,

> The epistemic burden of a course of action is everything a decision-maker must know (-that and -how), which they do not already know, in order to pursue the course of action effectively.

Those in power must realize that their position does not grant them any special abilities that allow them to know everything. Many decisions are made by officials in an office 10,000 miles away from the problem, surrounded by government officials who think and act in similar ways.

This individual has a far greater epistemic burden than the families and communities directly dealing with the issue. In this case, it would be wise to acknowledge that those closest to the issue are in a drastically better position to be able to understand the problems they face as well as the solutions.

Being able to understand the limits of one's capability to obtain knowledge about a problem is just as important as acquiring information.

Although the standard to decide to what extent policymakers are limited in their capacity to make a truly informed decision is unclear, a general inquiry into where that might be would go a long way. Likewise, society has greatly benefited from the general questioning of what the proper size of government should be rather than simply letting it run unhinged.

Instead of assuming politicians and bureaucrats to be all-knowing, there should be a robust debate of whether they are even in a position to understand what they are attempting to control.

For example, in attempting to contain the COVID-19 Pandemic, one can safely assume that a government official is knowledgeable enough to communicate some basic information regarding the virus. However, we should be incredibly skeptical of his or her ability to be knowledgeable enough to deem certain businesses essential and others non-essential. The information to make that decision belongs to the individual consumers and businesses that form a complex economic ecosystem.

On the futility of expecting policymakers to be informed enough to plan society Eric Nies writes,

> Planning as such is doomed to failure because of the insurmountable economic knowledge problem. As Frederick Hayek notes, "the 'data' from which the economic calculus starts are never for the whole society 'given' to a single mind which could work out the implications and can never be so given." Instead, you have numerous actors, each with incomplete knowledge, stepping on each other's feet.[340]

Both politicians and citizens must come to terms with the limits of their information and ability to make decisions on behalf of others. Scheall writes,

---

340 Nies, Eric. 2020. "COVID-19 and the Planners' Need to Plan." *Mises Institute*, March 26.

> Constituents might demand action of policymakers that the latter neither know of nor can learn enough to make effective… Even if surrogates have nothing but the interests of their surrogates in mind, their ignorance can prevent them from acting in ways that promote those interests.

When we empower governors to lock down their economies and implement phased reopening measures, we must also understand that those in power physically lack the ability to truly understand what they are attempting to control. Scheall explains,

> Policymakers are not gods. They are neither omniscient nor omnipotent. Their knowledge or relevant facts and theories is limited, as are their powers.

Nobody, not even supercomputers can even begin to comprehend the countless moving parts in society. This is why there have been disastrous unintended consequences from failing to understand informational limits.

There are few more guilty of hubris and ignorance than the epidemiologists and politicians who claim that millions would die if lockdowns were not instituted. Phil Magness explains how wildly incorrect some of the most influential experts were on predicting COVID-19 deaths.[341] He notes that,

> The Trump administration specifically cited ICL's 2.2 million death projection on March 16th when it shifted course toward a

341 Magness, Phillip W. 2020. "How Wrong Were the Models and Why?" *American Institute for Economic Research*, April 23.

> stringent set of "social distancing" policies, which many states then used as a basis for shelter-in-place orders.[342]

How can anyone be fit to not only understand a new virus that the medical community is still frantically researching but construct a model that can simulate the real-world consequences?

In this case, the experts and those in power did not know what they did not know. The 2.2 million death projection was wildly incorrect and the lockdown measures devastated the economy.

An article published by the Harvard Business Review warns that,[343]

> We still lack many of the basic facts about this disease, including how many people have symptoms, whether people who have been infected are immune to reinfection, and—crucially—how many people have been infected so far. In the absence of reliable virological testing data, we cannot fit models accurately, or know confidently what the future of this epidemic will look like for all these reasons, and yet numbers are being presented to governments and the public with the appearance of ccrtainty.[344]

---

342 Fink, Sheri. 2020. "White House Takes New Line After Dire Report on Death Toll." *The New York Times*, March 16.

343 Balsari, Satchit, Caroline Buckee and Tarun Khanna. 2020. "Which Covid-19 Data Can You Trust?" *Harvard Business Review*, May 8.

344 Bay, Jason. 2020. "Automated contact tracing is not a coronavirus panacea." *Medium*, April 10.

This goes to show the massive epistemic shortcomings of our response and mechanisms being employed against COVID-19. As leaders proclaim that they have all the answers to the crisis, this is a classic instance of not knowing what we don't know.

The article goes on the say that,

> Jason Bay, the product lead of Singapore's successful tracing app, TraceTogether, cautions that "automated contact tracing is not a coronavirus panacea." Yet some app-based contact-tracing efforts are being used to risk-stratify people, and these estimates are being used to make decisions on quarantine, isolation, and freedom of movement, without concomitant testing.

Contact tracing along with many other resources are oftentimes hailed as one of the government's magical tools to help combat COVID-19. However, by examining these mechanisms through an epistemological lens, we realize that they are incredibly ineffective at relieving policymaker ignorance.

Not only are things like contact tracing and epidemiological models highly imperfect, but the execution of nationwide policy requires knowledge that is simply unattainable at the macrolevel. Such missing knowledge includes information about the individual nuances of communities, how government policy will intersect with socioeconomic circumstances, and unintended consequences.

From an epistemological perspective, the government is not cutting with a scalpel, it's swinging a sledgehammer with a blindfold.

The problem of policymaker ignorance is something society often takes for granted. Although mocking politicians for poor decision-making and lack of knowledge is a common practice, Scheall's book shows that these problems are structural, not just individual.

Liberal democracies generally understand there are natural and just limits on the scope of government. The state cannot magically eliminate poverty with the stroke of a pen, nor does it have the right to silence our freedom of expression without losing its legitimacy.

In the pursuit of a more perfect union and better decision-making, we should begin to contemplate the epistemic limits of government. To inquire into the limits of knowledge acquisition and understanding. To what extent can those at the individual, local, state, and federal level act with an adequate understanding of the consequences of their actions and the needs of those they govern?

Scheall remarks at the end of his book that "There is a tradeoff between effective government and ambitious government."

Our experience with COVID-19 should be the catalyst for bringing epistemological inquiry into the mainstream discussion. There are plenty of debates to be had about the structural ignorance that is inherent to policymaking. What knowledge is accessible to decision-makers and what information is exclusive to the governed? Is the government even capable of understanding the full implications of shutting down the economy and closing schools? To what extent do public health experts truly have the tools and expertise to make the recommendations they make, with the degrees of certainty they employ?

At the moment the answer is unclear as epistemological inquiry has yet to become a mainstream discussion topic. However, coming to terms with what decision-makers can and cannot know will be a clear step in creating a more humble and effective government.

## PANDEMIC POLICY IN ONE PAGE

BY DAVID HART

May 29, 2020

Anybody who wishes to argue for a government monopoly which will "centrally plan" any industry or service (in this case public health during a pandemic) needs to come up with some very good reasons. So far, looking at both the theory and reality, I've seen no strong case for government to exercise monopoly controls during a pandemic, to say nothing for lockdowns, closures, travel bans, and controls on the population generally. Nothing about the presence of a virus, whether mild or severe, negates the problems with coercive central planning.

In fact, all the sound reasons why central planning does not and cannot work in the case of the general economy apply equally in this case, along with a few other reasons which are specific to epidemics.

Here are some of those reasons.

**1. The Knowledge Problem.** Central Planners need to know an almost infinite amount of knowledge concerning consumer demand, the resources controlled by producers, the level of prices, production processes, and the infinite variables of time and place. This they can never and will never have for good Hayekian reasons.[345]

Central Planners of Public Health need to know who is sick, where they are, how sick they are, what strain of the virus they are suffering from, what are their other physical conditions, what medical facilities

345 Carden, Art. 2019. "Read Hayek As If Your Children's Lives Depend On It." *American Institute for Economic Research*, May 10.

they have access to, how they will change their behaviour once they know they are sick, how they got sick, how to stop the spread, and what happens to the virus if it is stopped.[346]

The nightmare we have been watching unfold about the inadequate and often contradictory, and certainly partial information available to Central Planners of Public Health all over the world should be a warning to us that the knowledge problem here is as insurmountable as anything faced by the Stalinists and Maoists in the past.

**2. The Weakness of Mathematical Models.** It was a pipedream of the original Central Planners that computers would solve the knowledge problem, or at least make a good fist of processing the huge amount of data that governments and state managers had collected. This was never able to be put into practice because the amount of knowledge was too great (even for computers) and it kept changing faster than they could process it, and because the models they drew up were flawed and did not (could not) adequately describe how the economy worked.

The same is clearly the case with the mathematical models which have guided the decisions made by the Central Planners of Public Health. The Imperial College London models have had an abysmal track record going back nearly 20 years; their predictions have been astronomically wrong, and it is astonishing that they would have been used today to make such important decisions.[347] The incompetence of the data gatherers in the US and Europe is breathtaking, not to mention the dodgy data being given out by the Chinese government. How do

---

346 Viruses don't just disappear.

347 Magness, Phillip W. 2020. "How Wrong Were the Models and Why?" *American Institute for Economic Research*, April 23.

we (could we) know that any future Central Planners would do any better? Would they (could they) come up with a better model? I would say never in a million years.

**3. The One-Size-Fits-All Problem.** Given the national, regional, ethnic, behavioural, and climatic differences which exist (Hello! it was summer in Australia and not the winter flu season when all this began!) it is again not surprising that the "one size fits all" solution hasn't worked. It is always the first choice of the Central Planners because it is the most manageable one. If one wants to argue that the future Central Planners would allow more local solutions to be tried and implemented then it would no longer be a "central" plan or a (central) government monopoly, depending on how granular you wanted it to be.

For a "government" solution to the problem to work, what is the optimum geographical area for this to work: the "empire" (the US or the EU), the nation, the state, the region, the city (the big city or the small city?), the county, the street, the household? What the bumbling of the past couple of months has clearly revealed is that the solution which might suit Brooklyn in NYC is not suitable for the lakeshore town of Dunkirk in upstate NY.

**4. The Problem of Cost and Expenditure.** Like any Central Planner, Public Health Planners would not know what to spend what amount of money on what district to do what things or on/for whom, not to mention when to start and when to stop. They might say something as general as a "lockdown" or quarantining only the sick would not cost much, but anything beyond that becomes so complex and politicized as to be almost impossible to carry out. All sorts of public choice issues will (and have) occurred, such as Cuomo's political ambitions,

Trump's hubris, Fauci's reputation, pharmaceutical manufacturers, the high voting turnout of the elderly, Neil Ferguson's sex life, etc.[348] Not to mention the irrational panic among the general public fanned into flames by an irresponsible and ignorant mainstream media.

**5. The Problem of Unintended Consequences.** How do the Central Planners of Public Health calculate the cost-benefit analysis of their proposed measures? At present it seems they were too panicked to give this a second thought, or even if they had the thought to begin with (which I doubt). The all-seeing, all-knowing Planners would have to show how they could do this in a just and reasonable way, which I believe would be impossible to do. They would have to make calculations on how to spend scarce resources which might mean some officials (elected or appointed?) making some Benthamite calculation about who or what constitutes "the greatest number" and what their "greatest happiness" would look like.

As part of this calculation, you have to consider missed surgeries and medical appointments, deaths from suicide and drug overdoses, depression and famine in other parts of the world, far-reaching economic costs of shutting down businesses, layoffs, enforced isolation, ending freedom of movement, explosion in the debt, monetary expansion and resulting distortion, the "ratchet effect" of the increase in government

348 Stringham, Edward Peter. 2020. "Was Lockdown Architect and Theoretical Physicist Neil Ferguson Morally Right To Defy the Lockdown?" *American Institute for Economic Research*, May 18.

power, and other effects of the plan.[349]

**6. The Problem of Political Responsibility.** If there is one day a government monopoly in the provision of public health, will the Central Planners of Public Health be held legally liable for the mistakes they are bound to make? If their mathematical model of the epidemic is wrong, if the unintended consequences (the costs in money and lives lost) is worse than the disease, can they be sued in court for damages, or at least voted out of office if they are elected officials? Governments are not good at admitting error much less arranging compensation for the victims of their policies.

**7. The Problem of Individual Liberty.** I won't say more on this than state it. To me it seems rather obvious.

---

349 Tucker, Jeffrey A. 2020. "Lockdown Suicide Data Reveal Predictable Tragedy." *American Institute for Economic Research*, May 22; Salter, Alexander W. "Powell Admits that the Fed's Actions Vastly Exceed Its Mandate." *American Institute for Economic Research*, May 22.

# AFTERWORD

Everything from anthills to traffic patterns to slime molds to schools and herds of animals and cities are observed, studied, and analyzed for insights into how aggregates operate. The conditions under which living things move in lockstep, and the advantages they gain by doing so, are a fertile subcategory of study across both the physical and social sciences: within zoology, botany, microbiology, economics, sociology, and so on. The body collective dominates scientific inquiry.

But in every amassed group—even those with what barely passes for consciousness, at least from the human perspective—there are individuals that break away. They move outside, against, or in any event away from the community or prevailing trend: the bird that flees the flock, the bee that abandons the hive.

In the human world, and in particular the arts, outsiders tend to be celebrated. Writers, musicians, poets, painters, sculptors, and actors are so often misfits, and their creations embrace the plight and purpose of accidental or intentional nonconformists. Inventors, scientists, and other creators are at times notably eccentric, as were their forefathers, the shamans (some interesting speculation about whom is beyond the scope of this article) and healers.[350]

Across the spectrum of life, deviation from the norm occurs despite good reasons for flocking behaviors: efficiencies of scale, mutual protection, rudimentary information sharing, network benefits, and so on. But to borrow a programming adage: are mavericks a bug or a feature? After decades and perhaps centuries of discarding or ignoring them, science appears (however slowly) to be coming around to the study of outlier behavior. According to mathematical biologist Corina Tarnita of Princeton University:

> We spent a long time trying to understand how things synchronize. No one has really been [as] interested in the single cells that don't seem to do anything, or the lazy ants, or the wildebeests that for some reason decide not to migrate, or the locusts that peel off. We've just never really paid attention.[351]

Published in March 2020, just about when the lockdowns pursuant to the novel coronavirus pandemic began, Tarnita and team's PLoS paper "Eco-evolutionary significance of loners" ponders (albeit contextually): "Are loners incidental byproducts of large-scale coordination attempts,

---

350 Stern, David. 2012. "Masters of Ecstasy." *National Geographic*, December; Neilson, Susie. 2016. "A Mental Disease by Any Other Name." *Nautilus*, September 15; Carter, H. S. 1953. "Eccentrics in Medicine." *Glasgow Medical Journal*, 34(6): 259-269.

351 Cepelewicz, Jordana. 2020. "Out-of-Sync 'Loners' May Secretly Protect Orderly Swarms." *Quanta Magazine*, May 21.

or are they part of a mosaic of life-history strategies?"[352]

The article continues:

> Collective behaviors, in which a large number of individuals exhibit some degree of behavioral coordination, are frequent across the tree of life and across spatiotemporal scales: from microbial aggregates to the great wildebeest migration, from locust swarming to synchronized bamboo flowering, from fish schooling to mechanical adaptation in honeybee clusters. Intriguingly, however, such coordination is sometimes imperfect, and "out-of-sync" individuals (henceforth loners) have been reported in several of these systems. For instance, in locusts, population crowing prompts a transition from a solitary phase, in which in which individuals repel one another, to a gregarious phase, in which they attract each other. Experiments show, however, that not all individuals undergo this transition, even if exposed to long periods of crowding.

And it goes on elsewhere in the animal kingdom as well:

> In wildebeest, hundreds of thousands of individuals coordinate with each other and organize herding migrations, but resident populations that fail to migrate also exist. Similarly, wildebeest calving times are highly coordinated, but some fraction of the calves are born outside the calving period.

---

352 Rossine, Fernando W., Ricardo Martinez-Garcia, Allyson E. Sgro, Thomas Gregor, Corina E. Tarnita. 2020. "Eco-evolutionary significance of 'loners.'" *PLoS Biol* 18(3): e30000642.

Other research points in a similar direction.[353] Are these individuals and klatches a product of pure randomness, biological flukes, or cogs in a deeper evolutionary machine? Although that question has not been a scientific priority, there have been some empirical trailheads: "Theoretical investigations of such loner behaviors have been sparse, but the handful of existing studies have suggested that, at least in some systems, they could be a means of spatiotemporal niche partitioning that promotes diversity." There is no evidence that the propensity to idiosyncratic behavior is heritable, and thus "there exists no empirical evidence, in any system, that loners are anything more than chance stragglers[.]"

The authors go on to explain how in the cellular slime mold *Dictyostelium discoideum* (a strange and fascinating creature with the ability to convert from thousands of unicellular amoeba to a multicellular, slug-like creature) there are certain cells which do not, as the vast majority do, join in its multicellular life stage.[354] While in that state they remain "invulnerable to the threats of the multicellular stage but capable of reachieving multicellularity via their offspring," their behavior "may constitute insurance against such threats and therefore be critical" to the colony's survival. Broader still,

> [B]eyond multicellularity and sociality, [the] results have potential implications for the broadly analogous loner behaviors

353 Tarnita, Corina E., Alex Washburne, Ricardo Martinez-Garcia, Allyson E. Sgro, and Simon A. Levin. 2015. "Fitness tradeoffs between spores and non-aggregating cells can explain the coexistence of diverse genotypes in cellular slime molds." *PNAS*, 112(9): 2776-2781.

354 Wikipedia. 2020. "Dictyostelium discoideum." *Wikipedia*, July 27.

> identified across a variety of systems in which some form of coordination or synchronization is observed, from insects to vertebrates to plants. Our findings represent the first demonstration that loner behaviors can indeed . . . exhibit significant ecological consequences . . . While the mechanisms underlying the existence of loners are likely different across systems, the widespread existence of loners and the possibility that they could in fact be shaped by selection suggest an interesting conjecture: that, in general, imperfect coordination among individuals may enable evolution to shape population-partitioning strategies . . .and thus for system-level robustness.

It is of course possible to take conclusions far further than is warranted. And there is a vast difference between noisy gene expression, which can sometimes account for differences between otherwise identical individuals, and human choice. But a growing acceptance that individuals and small dissident clusters are consequential, and thus critical to holistic understanding of systems, is a huge step forward for scientific inquiry in the natural and social sciences.

Of particular importance to the topics covered in this book, there are hints that even computational approaches to the social sciences are at the cusp of embracing this awareness. As an interdisciplinary 2015 George Mason University master's thesis notes, with respect to agent-based models (ABMs),

> One value of ABMs is that they allow for collection of all details of the characteristics and behavior over time of every individual agent and the environment, theoretically enabling the analysis of micro-level interactions between individuals

> and within small groups. In practice, however, the volume of raw data generated by each run of a model (thousands of which might be done to test a range of parameters) makes it difficult to identify unusual interactions, and analysis of models ends up being done by aggregating data and reporting overall trends.[355]

And thus, as a corrective, the author discusses "using computer-generated narratives describing the behavior of an individual agent as an alternate method for evaluating the micro-level behavior of an ABM," and goes on to detail ways to identify and study "interesting" individual agents. Doing so may provide deeper insights or highlight flaws in the assumptions or design of economic, epidemiological, or any other such simulation.

In the meantime, it is jarring to think that highly-trained people - people who themselves tend toward independent and often iconoclastic thought - are late to arrive at the notion that individuals straying from a community may be nontrivial. The rogue elephant here, the person refusing to wear a mask there: perhaps intransigence, but perhaps responding to an arcane, numinous dictate beyond the explicitly knowable.

Computer models and simulations have fed fear and enlivened tyranny. Many millions of people in the real world continue to suffer and, indeed, die under pandemic policies wrought by the output of iteratively-run code. The scientific recognition of the social value of the asocial, in which our individual hopes, fears, personalities, and relationships are no longer assumed away or subsumed by mathematical

355 Auble, Brent D. 2015. "Narrative Agents as a Reporting Mechanism for Agent-Based Models." *George Mason University.*

averages, is a subtle but monumental breakthrough. Here's hoping it continues.

**Peter C. Earle**

July 29, 2020

# ABOUT THE EDITOR

Peter C. Earle is an economist and writer who joined AIER in 2018 and prior to that spent over 20 years as a trader and analyst in global financial markets at a number of firms and funds.

His research focuses on financial markets, monetary policy, virtual and cryptocurrencies, and issues in economic measurement. He has been quoted in *The Wall Street Journal*, *Bloomberg*, *Grant's Interest Rate Observer*, *Reuters*, *NPR*, and in numerous other publications.

Pete holds an MA in Applied Economics from American University, an MBA (Finance), and a BS in Engineering from the United States Military Academy at West Point.

# ABOUT AIER

The American Institute for Economic Research in Great Barrington, Massachusetts, was founded in 1933 as the first independent voice for sound economics in the United States. Today it publishes ongoing research, hosts educational programs, publishes books, sponsors interns and scholars, and is home to the world-renowned Bastiat Society and the highly respected Sound Money Project. The American Institute for Economic Research is a 501c3 public charity.

Printed in Great Britain
by Amazon

71646923R00166